ONE
TWO
PUNCH™

by Claudia Wilson, MS, RDN, CSSD, CSCS

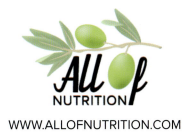

WWW.ALLOFNUTRITION.COM

Copyright © 2018 by Claudia Wilson

All rights reserved. This book or any portion thereof may not be reproduced or used in any manner whatsoever without the express written permission of the publisher except for the use of brief quotations in a book review.

Printed in the United States of America

First Printing, 2018

ISBN 978-1717049216

www.allofnutrition.com

ONE TWO PUNCH™

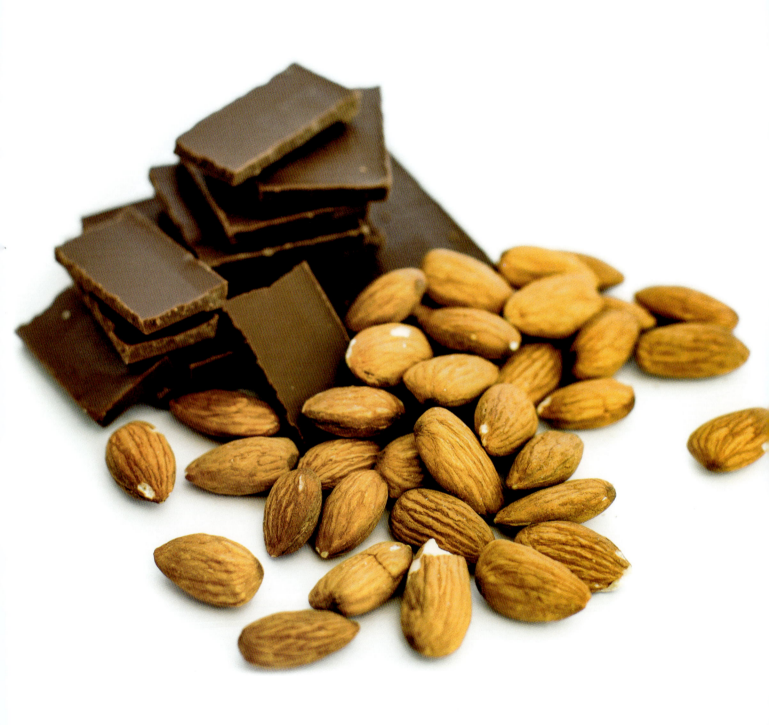

TABLE OF CONTENTS

INTRODUCTION 1

Eating Influences 5

BURN 13

The Incinerator 15

Incinerator Graph 17

Partly Cloudy or…. "Clear as Mud" 23

Deciding Hunger Graph 33

Hydrate the Incinerator 34

Water Guidelines 35

Water in the ONE-TWO PUNCH 36

Rest the Incinerator 37

BALANCE 41

The Protein Anchor 43

Blood Sugar Graph 45

ONE-TWO PUNCH 48

Nut Chart 52

Legume Chart 56

Milk Chart 58

Carbohydrate Foods 63

Protein Foods	65
Hybrid Foods	67
Mixed Foods	69
Fats	71
Portion Distortion	74
Plate Graph	75
Permission	76
"The Devil is in the Details"	87

BECOME — 91

Practice Hunger	98
Hunger/Fullness Scale	98
Hunger Gauge	100
How to Respond to Physical Hunger	103
Meal Plans	104
Practice Emotions	107
Types of Hunger	109
Practice with Fullness	115
Non-Distracted Eating	115
Paced Eating	116
Feeling Chart	120

Practice without Training Wheels ... 121

And Practice Some More ... 121

CONCLUSION — 125

Burn ... 128

Balance ... 128

Become ... 128

FAQ — 132

What if I'm still hungry after a balanced fist each of protein and carbohydrate? ... 133

Do I need to change this plan if I exercise? ... 133

Why isn't fat counted? ... 133

When should I have breakfast? ... 133

Is there a time that is too late to eat? ... 134

What's the difference between a meal and a snack? ... 134

What should I do when I eat out? ... 135

What if I hate vegetables? ... 135

Can I follow this method if I have diabetes? ... 135

Where does diet soda fit? ... 137

Can I eat with other people and still practice mindful eating? ... 137

How can I do this while traveling? ... 137

Will I lose weight while following this?	137
How is this better than intuitive eating?	137
Can I do this while taking medication?	137
Is this okay to do while pregnant or nursing?	138
Should I weigh myself while doing this? How often?	138
What if I gain weight?	138
What supplements and vitamins should I take?	140
How many fruits and vegetables should I eat during the day?	140
Can my kids do this with me?	140
What if I am vegetarian or vegan?	140
Can I do this together with another plan like Paleo™ or Whole30™?	140
Should I buy organic foods?	140

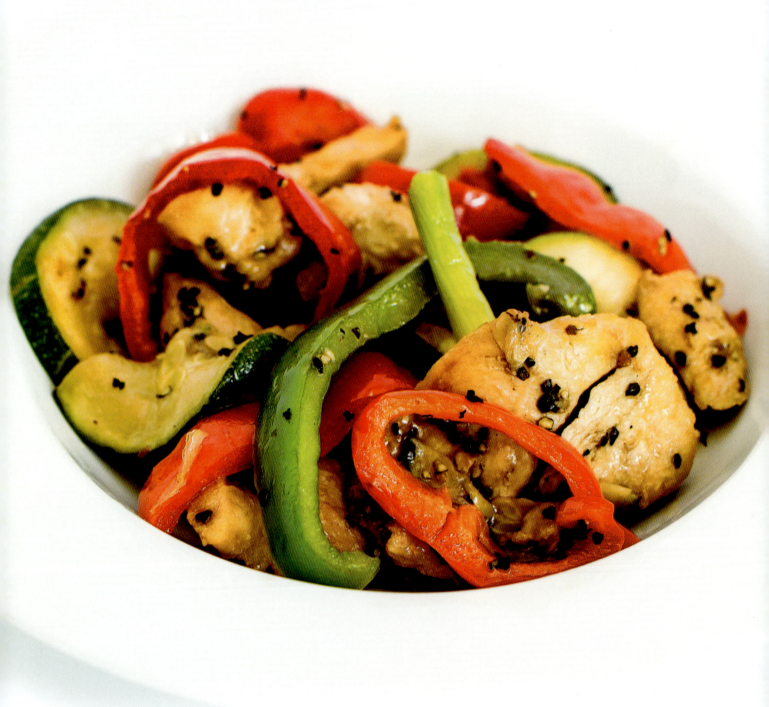

INTRODUCTION

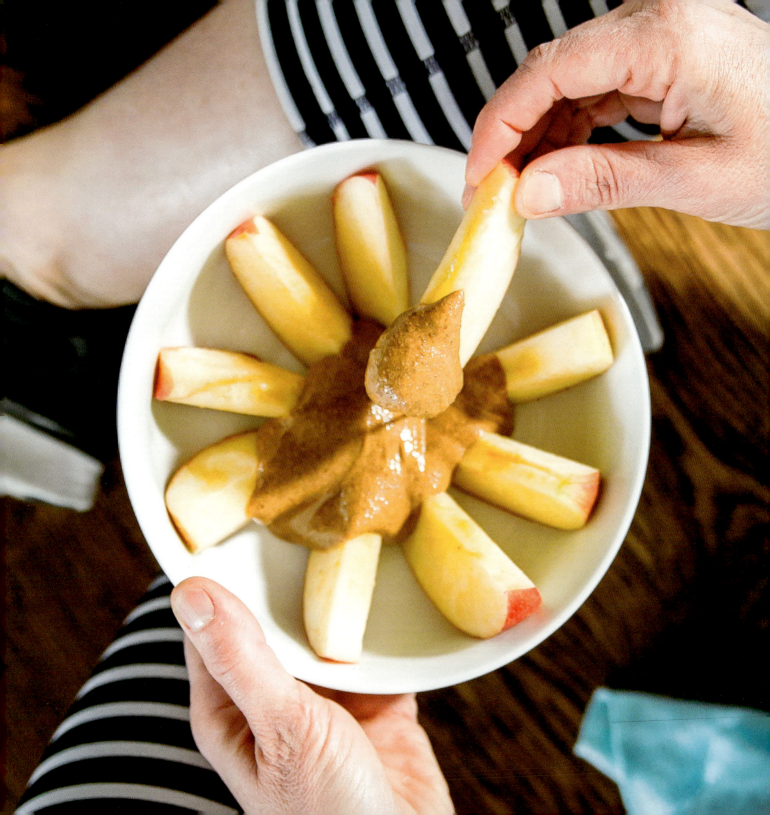

Do you want to eat healthy without trying too hard? Are you tired of dieting to get the results you want? Why is it so complicated? Why do we need so many plans, directions, instructions and laws governing our eating? Every year it is something different. Eat this, don't eat that! Oh wait, scratch that! Well, let's see. Okay, hold please for more research. Is that how you feel? We are spending billions of dollars on programs and products, yet not becoming healthier as a society or as individuals.[1-4]

I agree that eating healthy can feel complex. However, I don't think it needs to be complicated or confusing. This book shows you how to make it SIMPLE, UNDERSTANDABLE and DOABLE — without measuring, without counting, without tracking, without eating special foods and without stressing.

During my 20 years of practice, I have found that some individuals struggle with the concept of intuitive and mindful eating. It feels too vague, too abstract and more like free-falling.

Maybe it's because of our society's increasing emphasis on "eating within the lines" or our increasing anxiety to do things right in a world and culture that has become increasingly more focused on perfection and achievement. Whatever the reasons, I discovered that individuals needed some structure WITHIN the parameters of intuitive and mindful eating and my purpose is to provide this structure. But I don't want to abandon the idea that we can learn or re-learn how to recognize hunger and respond to it in a way that is physically and emotionally nourishing and sensually satisfying.

I am determined to provide a structured and flexible way to eat. And do it without restriction and without dieting, measuring, tracking or eating special foods. I'll recommend when to eat, what to eat and how to make it sustainable.

You can practice this method in any city, any country, any restaurant and at any age. This is ONE-TWO PUNCH.

ONE-TWO PUNCH (OTP) was specifically created to show you how to put the best aspects of nutrition information into action — in a way that makes sense. It's designed to feel comfortable and still allow you to reach your health and fitness goals.

This concept evolved as I was trying to simplify food and eating for individuals visiting with me. There are so many things influencing our behavior with food. Without help, it can be overwhelming.

Plain and simple, I am an EATING COACH. Every day I coach individuals to improve their relationship with food; to help them understand, recognize and honor their body cues while also trying to sort out the confusion about the nutrition advice coming at them every day.

Groundbreaking and sensational work on this concept was introduced by Evelyn Tribole and Elyse Resch in their first book, Intuitive Eating. Many Registered Dietitian Nutritionists (RDNs) refer to this book as "the bible" when it comes to an emotionally healthy relationship with food.

Let me review a couple of definitions. Intuitive eating includes rejecting the dieting mentality, using nutrition information without judgment and respecting your body, regardless of how you feel about its shape. Intuitive eating summarily is the practice of eating for physical rather than emotional reasons, relying on internal hunger and satiety cues and the unconditional permission to eat.[5-6] Mindful eating is a process of paying attention to your actual eating experience, without judgment.[6-8] Aspects of both intuitive eating and mindful eating are used throughout this book.[9-11]

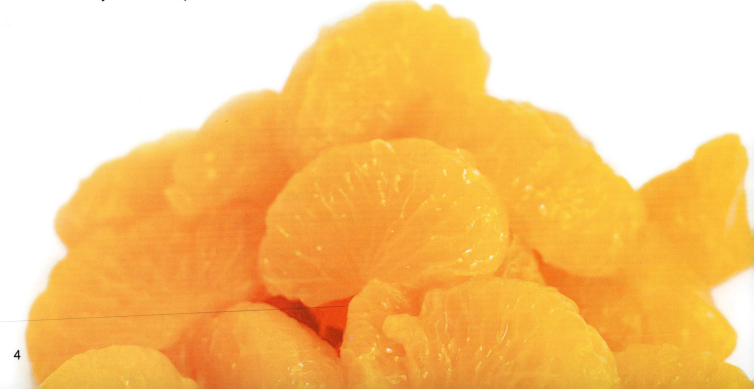

Eating Influences

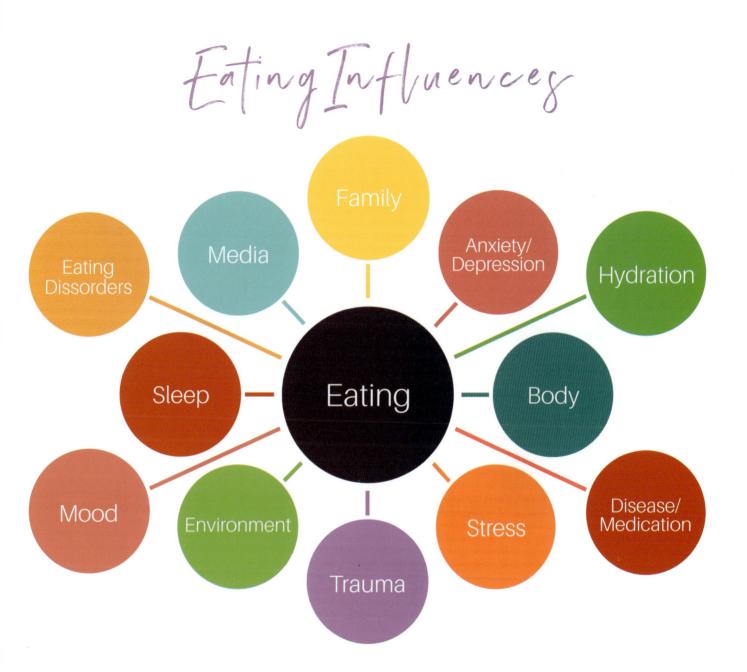

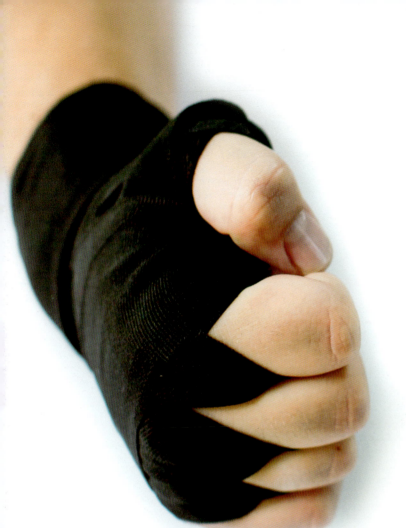
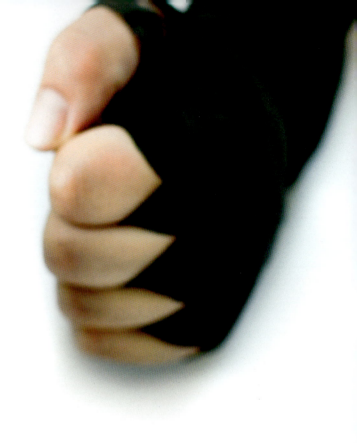

Eat when your body will **BURN** it
BALANCE what you eat
BECOME the YOU you've always wanted

This book is for you if...

- You want to be healthy and fit without trying too hard.

- You are tired of dieting, with the accompanying tracking, counting, measuring.

- You want to be healthier, but don't know where to start.

- You get discouraged after falling "off the wagon."

- You feel defeated after a cheat meal.

- You've tried diet after diet, only to gain the weight back and then some.

- You feel that eating healthy is too complicated.

- You don't have the time or energy to eat healthy.

- You want a program that you can do for the rest of your life.

- You want to be able to eat with friends and family without feeling deprived.

This could be you!

Finally...something has clicked in my psyche after a lifelong battle with weight and food obsession. After a lot of therapy, cultivating my spirituality and my work with Claudia, I'm probably the happiest I've ever been in my life. I am 36 years old and have been on diets since I was 7. I obsessed over food and dieting, the scale, what I ate and who saw me eat it. Finally, I don't feel controlled by food. I feel empowered and know how to fuel and take care of my body and my soul.

When I first started working with Claudia, I felt hopeless, powerless and out of control. I thought if I could lose weight, everything would be fine, I would feel in control. So, naturally I booked a visit with a dietitian. I was hoping she would tell me what to eat and when and put me on a calorically-calculated meal plan. She did none of that. In our first visit her primary recommendation was to get some sleep! Best. Advice. Ever.

When I was better rested, we moved on to talking about my relationship with food and my emotional triggers that lead to eating. We worked on my awareness of hunger and fullness, and although I felt I failed again and again at recognition, she assured me that I was indeed learning and making progress.

I had no idea Claudia would help me completely change the way I thought about food, myself and my own power. She also recommended I start seeing a therapist. Through our continued work she helped normalize a lot of my eating behaviors and helped me understand my shame patterns with eating. She helped me understand why I felt compelled to eat when I was feeling powerless in my life.

I was anxious about trusting myself with my feelings and food. I literally did not feel like I had the power to eat when I was hungry and stop when I was full. Binge eating ice cream in a hot bath was my sanctuary after a stressful lonely day. I didn't want my only way to decompress taken away. Binging felt like a long deep breath. I used food to make me feel good and to numb my feelings of powerlessness. Ironically, it intensified my powerlessness by making me feel sick and overweight.

I worked hard to understand my interactions with food, challenging 30 years of core beliefs related to food and worthiness. I learned that I'm loveable no matter how much I weigh or how much I eat. I learned I needed to take care of my psychological and spiritual health before I could even begin to figure out how to be at peace with food. I learned to be compassionate with myself and relax about my food choices.

I now feel empowered to eat when I'm hungry and stop when I'm full. I slowly learned that when I eat a fist of protein with a fist of carbs I stay full longer and don't crash. And, it's curbed my sweet tooth. I have stopped mindlessly eating. I am not obsessed about thinking of food and what type of food, and when I'm going to get it. My eating is a process, not a destination. After all my hard work, I now feel so much peace.

-Lindsey

Disclaimer

This method is not going to solve everyone's issues with food. It's just not. That's my preamble to all the naysayers that will say this isn't complicated enough. Seriously? This is not a detailed, quick fix plan. It doesn't have a lot of bells and whistles. It won't help you lose 10 pounds in a week. It may not help you lose 20 pounds in a month, but you will improve your relationship with food and your body. It is going to take effort and thought, even though it is simple. It will require a lifestyle and mind shift in your relationship with all food. And it is going to require trust. Trust in the information found in this book and trust in yourself. It is a long-term, sustainable, do-anywhere, at any-age plan. It does take work. It does take commitment. Apply this method and don't overanalyze it. Think about the bigger issues of your life like friends, family, work and so on.

Pay attention to your body's physical hunger—BURN. Combine key nutrients every time you eat—BALANCE. ONE-TWO PUNCH will help you BECOME a healthy weight and have a healthy relationship with food. Let's get started!

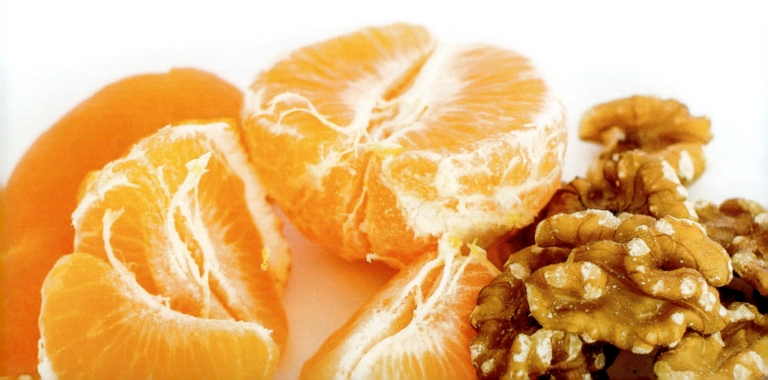

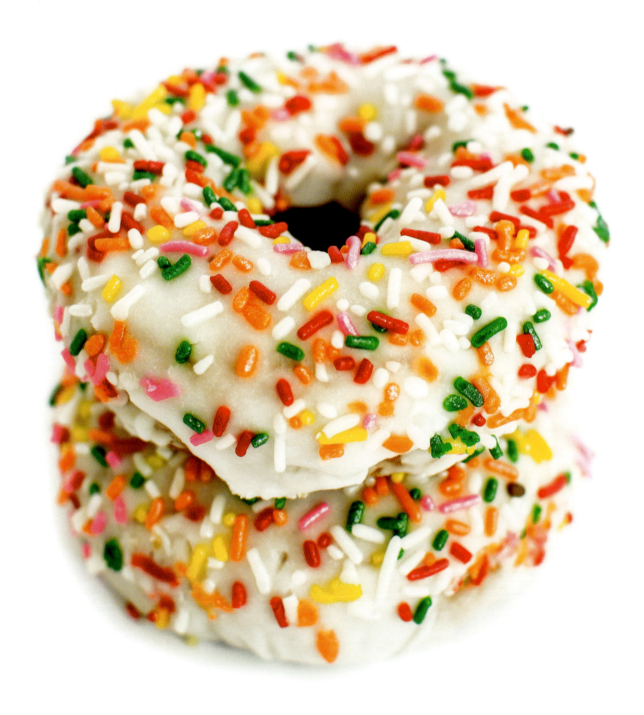

BURN

The first and most crucial part of ONE-TWO PUNCH is BURN: eating when you are hungry. Even if you stop doing any other part of ONE-TWO PUNCH, keep adhering to the foundational principle of eating when you are hungry. Recognizing physical hunger and eating when you feel that sensation is the foundation you continually return to through this process.

Physical hunger can be difficult to detect. When your body needs food you may start to feel weak, tired or feel a lack of concentration. Your stomach may start to ache and rumble. If your hunger continues your stomach may start to really hurt and you may find it more difficult to concentrate. You may also feel lightheaded and nauseous. Some people get shaky and feel nervous, while others start to get a headache.

All of us feel hunger differently, in ways that are unique to us.[8-9] Even in the same person it might feel different at different times. For example, when I get hungry in the morning, my stomach rumbles; when I feel hunger in the afternoon, it's sometimes a painful sensation.

THE INCINERATOR

Think of your stomach as an incinerator. An incinerator is a machine for burning materials at high temperatures. The materials are placed in the incinerator through an open door that can be closed when it is full. In this analogy I want you to think of the material as food. When you feel hungry, it means the incinerator door is open. When you are full, the incinerator door is closed. More on fullness later.

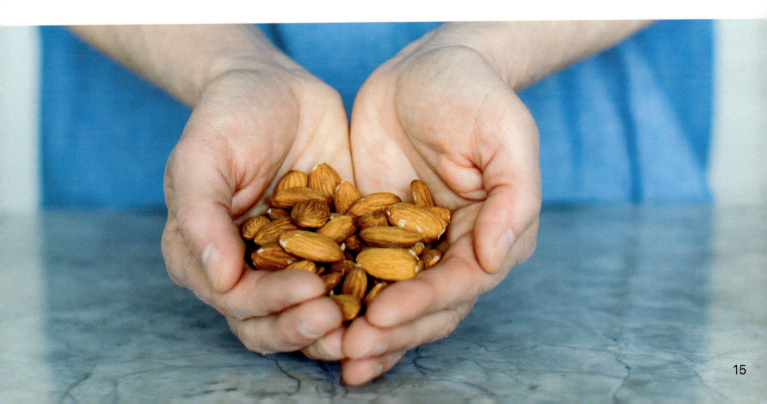

The incinerator, your stomach, will burn anything you put into it WHEN the door is open – anything! Yes, yes, of course, different foods are going to be burned at different rates, but remember we are trying to be UNCOMPLICATED. Anything you put in an incinerator with an open door is going to be burned.

Scientifically, when you are hungry your body secretes ghrelin, the hunger hormone, to signal your need to eat.[14-20] When your body produces ghrelin, you get hungry and your incinerator door opens. Anything that you put inside is going to be burned.[15,17]

As you eat, your stomach is stretched and the secretion of ghrelin stops. As ghrelin stops, the incinerator door begins to close - very, very slowly. REALLY slowly! It truly takes 20 to 30 minutes for your brain to register fullness as it receives signals from the filling stomach.[21-23] Leptin is the fullness hormone. It regulates food intake by signaling fullness.[15,17,19-20]

Leptin kicks in to signal that it is time to stop eating. The more leptin produced, the fuller you feel.[15,19,21,24] Leptin is like the door closing on the incinerator to tell you when it is time to stop eating.[14-15,25-26]

For the purpose of this book and to decrease confusion, I am over-simplifying a complex process. In a way, ghrelin and leptin act in opposition to each other for the body to maintain ideal energy balance or ideal body weight.[15,19,26] But being the complicated humans that we are, this system has many loopholes.[16,27-28]

The incinerator, your stomach, can only burn and process so much food at a time. OF COURSE, you can override or trick the closing door of the incinerator. This happens when you eat super fast, like in less than 5 minutes, and you eat enough to feed a family of four without even realizing what you are doing. And THEN the door closes 20 minutes later. Remember, I said it closes very slowly.

ghrelin = HUNGER = open door
(think of grrrr, stomach growling for ghrelin)

leptin = FULLNESS = closed door
(think of fullllll, up to your lips for leptin)

THE INCINERATOR

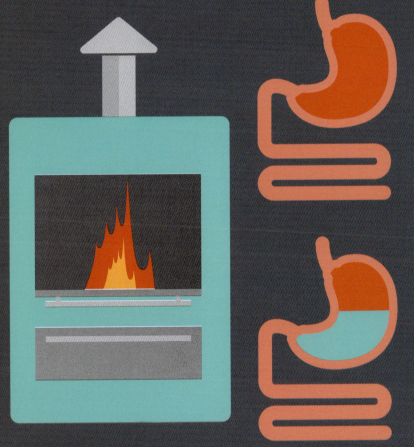

An incinerator is a device that burns waste and reduces it to ash. When the incinerator is turned on and the door is open, anything you throw in there is going to be burned.

An empty stomach signals the body to secrete a hormone called ghrelin that creates hunger. When you feel hunger, your body is ready to burn what you put in it.

As you eat, the secretion of ghrelin gradually stops. Leptin takes over and signals that it is time to stop eating by making you feel full.

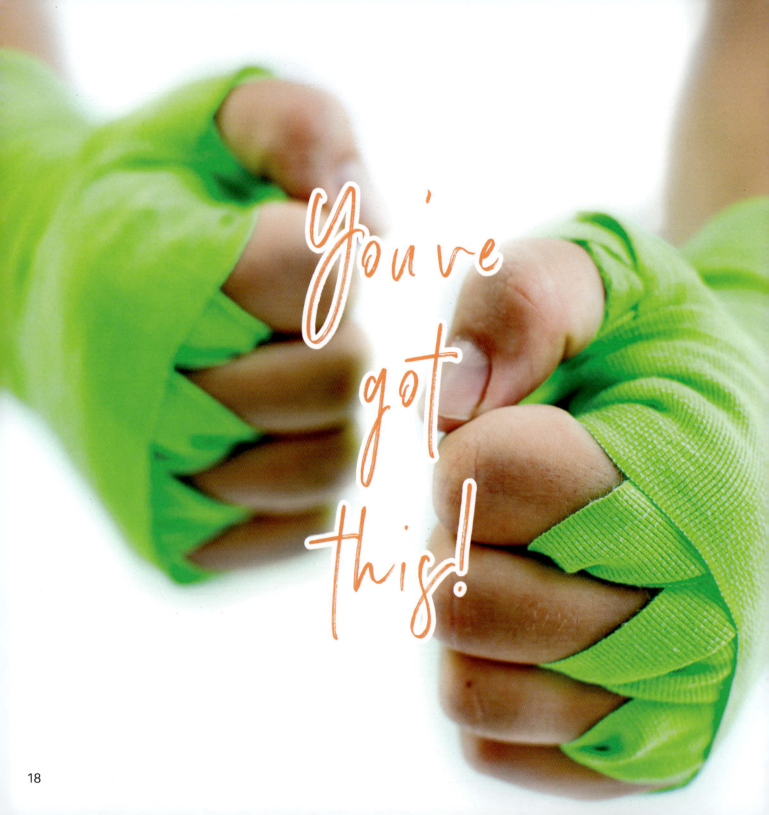

When you eat that quickly, you've tried to pack in much more food than the incinerator can actually handle. We've all done it and felt that, "Oooohhhhh, I feel so full; I went way too far" feeling. Why didn't your body tell you? Probably because you raced against the door and WON!!! Even if you aren't eating fast, you are a human with a smart brain. You can override, trick or ignore the system any time you want.

The human body has the capacity to eat way more than it can burn. And it has a compensation mechanism for every time you eat more than you can burn. It's a kind of storage channel to account for overeating — it's called fat storage.[29] You can eat more than the body needs before the door closes or you can ignore that the door has closed and keep eating.[30-31]

Ideally, we would all stop when we feel full, regardless of what we are eating. However, for lots of reasons, we keep eating, and eating and eating overriding the ghrelin/leptin system. We can continue to eat long after the door has closed. At this point your body says, "What am I going to do with this excess? I didn't need all this food and can only handle so much at one time. I guess I'll just use that compensation mechanism and store it for later." The incinerator does not change its capacity.[32]

When you eat on a "closed-door" incinerator, you have much more potential to store the extra food as fat. This is true of all foods whether it is a carbohydrate, protein or fat.[33] The incinerator cannot burn food sitting outside the closed door. The same thing happens when you eat when you aren't hungry, when the incinerator door didn't open. It is as if the food sits on top of a closed door, waiting to be stored. When it sits outside of a closed door, it has more potential to be stored as fat rather than wait around until the door opens again.[16,27-28]

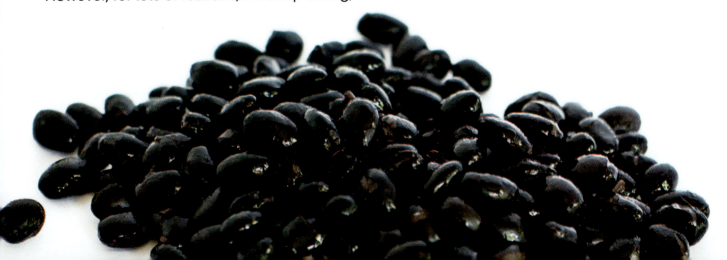

Unless something has gone metabolically[29] or genetically wrong, all humans are equipped with the mechanisms to signal hunger and fullness. However, there are conditions and circumstances that mask these mechanisms. Some of these reasons include eating disorders, diseases, medications, mood and our environment.[13,34]

Many things can confuse your ability to detect true physical hunger and fullness. If you've been ignoring your hunger and fullness signals for a while, your physical sensitivity to them decreases.[13] This comes from chronically restricting food intake, continually cleaning your plate or limiting eating to certain times when following a diet.

Here is what's super interesting about following a diet plan — how do you feel when you are trying like crazy to follow it? How do you feel when you're counting, tracking, measuring, reading, calculating and following directions? You feel STRESSED, right?!?! You think you're doing something good for your body by being on the program, but you're actually increasing your stress and increasing your cortisol.[35-36]

Cortisol is a steroid hormone made in the adrenal glands of the body. It is often called the stress hormone due to its connection to your stress response. Some research shows that a high level of cortisol may lead to weight gain.[35-36] You need to do something different. ONE-TWO PUNCH is different and easy to follow without increasing stress.

> Stress clouds your ability to sense true physical hunger or fullness and the cortisol cues your body to hang onto the fat.

Stress clouds your ability to sense true physical hunger or fullness, and the cortisol cues your body to hang onto the fat. So you're getting a double whammy. It's stressful to try to stay on a diet plan. On top of that, the increase in cortisol[35-36] is actively working against what you're trying to do!

If you've been following various diets for a long time, it may take practice to rediscover your hunger and fullness cues.[12-13] Your stomach comes to expect food at certain times. If you're in the habit of grazing all day, your body has been taught to crave a continual supply of food.

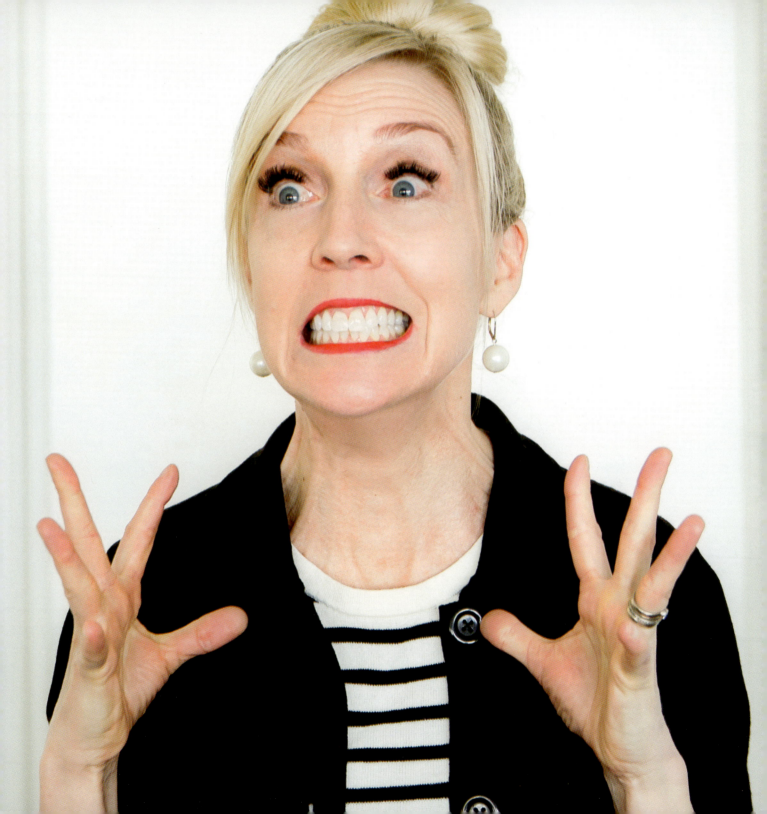

Hunger is your body's need to eat.

Appetite is the desire to eat.

It takes practice to recognize what physical hunger is as opposed to what else it might be. And remember, hunger can show itself in various ways. We all feel hunger differently, although there are generally recognized sensations.[13]

PARTLY CLOUDY OR.... "CLEAR AS MUD"

There are many things that can be mistaken for hunger. Your ability to detect hunger and fullness gets clouded by other influences; a primary influence is emotions. Any emotion under the sun can mask your sense of hunger. Stress is a term possibly used to describe ANY uncomfortable feeling. More specific words to describe stress might be anxiety, worry, sadness, anticipation, restlessness, frustration and loneliness. When any of these stressful emotions come up it can make you feel hungry when you are not.

Happy emotions can be confused with hunger too: excitement, anticipation, joy and love. All these emotions happen at your core. They catch you in your gut. That's where you feel them.

The ability to detect physical hunger and fullness can get blocked by any emotion, even happy, positive emotions. You feel the sensation of emotion in the center of your body, the same place you feel physical hunger.[37]

It is not just emotions that get in the way of detecting hunger and fullness. There are external triggers in your surrounding enviroment that make you believe you are hungry. Seeing and smelling food, especially yummy favorites, can make you think you are hungry. Really, what has increased is your appetite, not your physical hunger.[14,32,38-40]

Hunger is your body's need to eat, a compelling need for food.[14] If you're hungry, you need food because your body is telling you so by sending you signals. These signals can be painful, annoying and sometimes rumbling sensations, or a weakness you feel

> We CAN learn to control and change the level of our appetite. It takes practice to understand what triggers your appetite and what contributes to your hunger being confused by emotions.

over your entire body. Hunger cannot be dictated; it is instinctive.[41]

Appetite is the desire to eat, a fondness for or liking a particular food. Appetite is a coordinated effort between your brain and your stomach.[14] When you see a food that looks particularly tasty, your mouth may water. When this happens you can practically taste it and feel the textures in your mouth.

Even thinking about food can elicit the same response. But unlike hunger, appetite can be controlled. Your brain greatly influences appetite levels and your response to it. It is a learned behavior.[13-14] I know, now your brain is saying, "What???????" It's a little mind-blowing.

We CAN learn to control and change the level of our appetite. It takes practice to understand what triggers your appetite and what contributes to your hunger being confused by emotions.

Wanting a food, versus needing it, is a craving. Cravings are usually driven by appetite, very often an external cue. You want or crave a food after seeing it or thinking about it. Being at the checkout counter at Home Depot and seeing your favorite treat and wanting it as you buy duct tape is an external cue, not an internal cue (physical hunger).[13-14,40]

There are millions of external cues. Television commercials are a prime example.[14,39] That luscious, dripping burger that you weren't thinking of five minutes earlier, suddenly sounds pretty tasty. Part of this process, the work and commitment part, will require distinguishing physical hunger (an internal cue) from other appetite triggers (external cues).[14,38,42]

An external cue for many people is the clock. What makes you reach for something to eat? Do you feel the need to eat at "breakfast time" or "lunch time" or another typical mealtime? I frequently ask clients what prompts them to eat at a particular time. A common response is, "Because it's time for breakfast or because it's time for lunch." When I ask them about whether or not they were hungry, they're not sure.

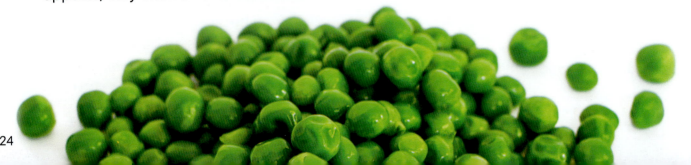

Mealtime is when your incinerator door is open.

It's a habit for many to eat breakfast in the morning at a designated time, without regard to what's happening in their body. And the importance of breakfast has been drilled into our heads for many years. Breakfast is an important meal, but so is every meal when you're hungry and the body needs fuel. It needs to be the first time you get hungry in the morning. For some people it might not be until they have been awake for a couple hours.

Do you think you're hungry when the clock strikes noon? Eating at "lunch time" when your body isn't asking for fuel increases your potential for fat storage. [43] My suggestion of breaking this pattern turns everything on its head.

If you have dieted chronically, your hunger and fullness signals may not be ideal and you'll need to slowly progress towards relying on your internal cue of hunger rather than the time on the clock. When mealtime hits, you can use it as a reminder to check in with your stomach and assess your hunger instead of automatically eating because it's time.

What I'm trying to emphasize in ONE-TWO PUNCH is that mealtime is when your incinerator door is open, utilizing your internal cue of physical hunger, not an external cue of the time on the clock. It's going to take practice to ignore the clock and focus instead on your stomach.

I believe if everyone could aptly detect their hunger and fullness (when the incinerator door is OPEN and when it is CLOSED) and eat accordingly, most people would be at appropriate weights and have

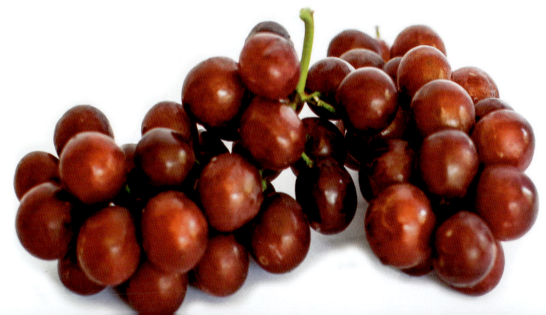

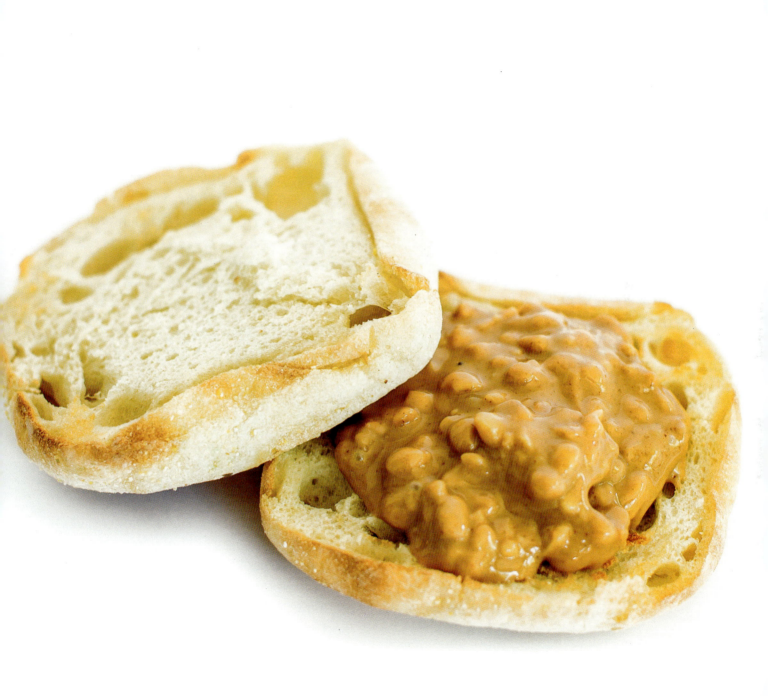

an appropriate relationship with food. Of course, there would still be a range of body types and sizes.

It is easy, so very easy, to mistake all kinds of other sensations for physical hunger. Because of that, it's also easy to eat for lots of reasons other than physical hunger.

Ideally, you are waiting for an internal physical stomach signal to grab you, interrupt you and pull you from what you are doing. Your hunger should knock at your door, not have you continually checking in with it. You shouldn't have to repeatedly ask, "Am I hungry now? How about now?" It will tell you.

When you ignore hunger or fullness, or if you don't recognize hunger or fullness, the incinerator is disregarded entirely.[13,44] The great news is you can learn or relearn how to distinguish physical hunger from appetite.

You can ask yourself whether your body indeed needs fuel. External sources of false hunger, like appetite and craving triggers, are usually for something specific, something delicious.

You can ask yourself, "Am I so hungry that I'd eat steamed broccoli, brown rice and grilled chicken?" If you're not actually physically hungry, chances are these won't sound inviting. When you're learning or relearning how to sense physical hunger, there's a series of steps you can take, one at a time, to increase your awareness of what's happening when you think you're hungry. It will take practice.

> Am I so hungry that I'd eat steamed broccoli, brown rice and grilled chicken?

The practice can sometimes be tedious because the essence of practice is repetition. You will need to practice detecting your physical hunger again and again.

The very next time you reach for something to eat or have the thought that you're hungry and need to seek out food, STOP. Pause for a minute before following through with the momentum of the moment and grabbing food. It helps in this moment to take a breath; one long, expansive breath. The breath alone can interrupt the mindless action of eating without really thinking about it.

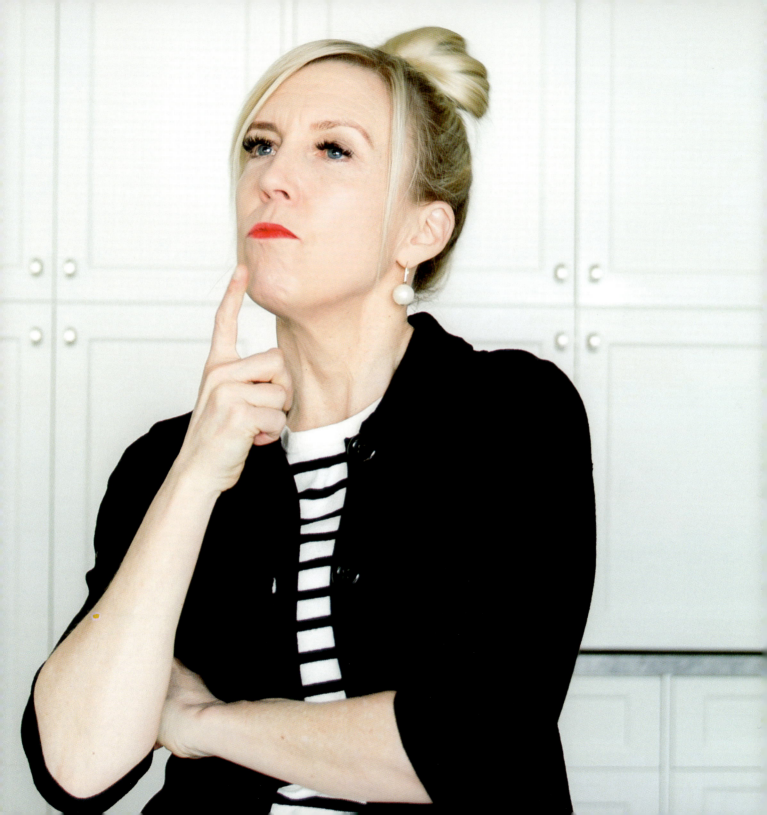

This could → be you!

I was raised in a clean-your-plate culture with media touting 5'10" female models weighing 106 pounds. My tall slender grandmother called me out as "pudgy" whenever I gained 5 pounds or more. I started dieting around age 14 and have yo-yoed my 5'5" body between 118 – 170 pounds too many times to count.

At age 44 and 169 pounds, I hired a personal trainer to successfully lose 35 pounds and lean down to 16% body fat by eating less and moving more. I ate very clean, finding ways to eat deliciously with no white flour, no white sugar, lots of fresh fruits and vegetables, whole grains, lean protein and some dairy.

I was happy my body had settled at a comfortable weight. But I had a lot of anxiety and fear around food in trying to maintain that weight. I controlled the anxiety by carefully monitoring macros and logging food intake most days. Within two years, I gained just 3 pounds and panicked. Eating less and moving more didn't take off the added weight, so I tried every other sensible diet: carb cycling, calorie cycling, calorie restriction + 2 cheat meals per week, intermittent fasting, smaller frequent meals and so on. I tried eating more as my trainer suggested. I threw science in the mix with body composition, VO2Max and RMR tests to predict how many daily calories I could consume to maintain my weight.

Exhausted, I came to Claudia for a formula I could program into my day to eliminate the burden of constantly monitoring and worrying about the effects of food. I expected she would help me calculate a calorie goal, develop a food plan and work with me to monitor changes. She instead taught me ONE-TWO PUNCH. More panic! I was so fearful to trust my hunger as a cue to eat. Part of my eating strategy was not to feel hunger to avoid "hangry" comments from friends and family.

With patience and practice, I embraced OTP. It became a relief to know how to respond to hunger. The most difficult part was recognizing my own fullness cues. For me, I stop eating when it is no longer satisfying or pleasurable. I can leave food on my plate without guilt. I learned I ate when I wasn't hungry, which I always thought was okay, because I was staying within a certain caloric limit.

Now I know I needed something besides food at those times. When I feel like turning to the cupboard and I'm not hungry, I take a 20-minute cat nap or drink a refreshing herbal tea or listen to a podcast. I fully enjoy many pleasures including food. I knew I mastered OTP when I returned from a week-long cruise and instead of gaining 5 pounds, I had lost weight. No more diets or daily calorie monitoring – I am finally at peace. I've maintained my weight now for years with OTP and concentrate more on my life than food.

—Suzanne

What's going on in your stomach? Are you having physical signs of hunger? If you're not sure what you are feeling physically have a large glass of water. I suggest 16 ounces of water. If you are truly physically hungry and not just thirsty, your physical sensations of hunger will return in 5-10 minutes.

What are you feeling and thinking at this point? If you think you're feeling physical signs of hunger are you willing to eat anything? Or is it specifically the donuts that someone brought into work today? If you are not yet feeling physically hungry, try to stay in this space and explore why you want something to eat. If you are indeed feeling physically hungry, forge ahead! Your incinerator door is open and your body will burn what you put inside.

Learn more about decipering physical hunger and what to do when you are NOT hungry in the BECOME section of this book.

Appetite, cravings, emotions and external cues influence your ability to detect hunger. There are two more things that GREATLY influence your ability to detect physical hunger and the signals coming from your incinerator.

Maintaining a car, bicycle or other type of machinery affects how it functions. There are two things that affect how your body incinerator functions: how much water you drink and how much sleep you get.

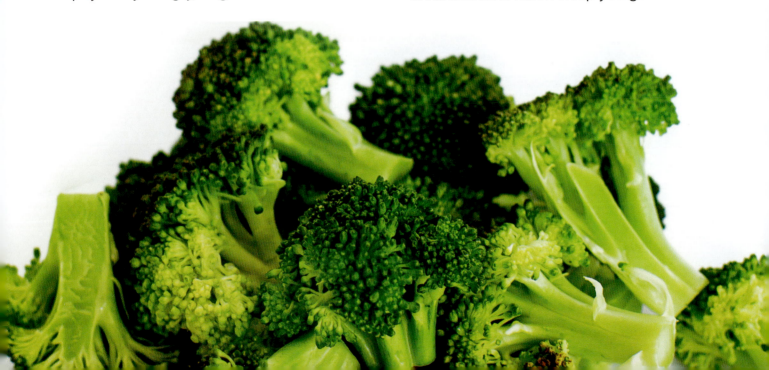

It all starts when you reach for something to eat. When you do, follow these steps:

 STOP Pause right where you are. Roll your shoulders all the way back (imagine a peacock strutting). BREATHE one full breath.

 ASK How do you feel? What are you physically feeling? What's going on emotionally?

 DRINK Drink about 16oz of water.

 WAIT Wait 10 minutes.

 ASK How do you feel now?

 ASK What are you reaching for? Why that? Would you still be hungry if your option was steamed broccoli?

 DECIDE YES OR NO
YES - Sensations are coming from your stomach; you're feeling empty.
NO - None of the sensations are really coming from your stomach.

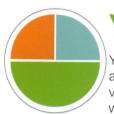 **YES | EAT** You're likely hungry. Choose a 🤜 protein and a 🤜 carbohydrate with 1/2 plate of veggies that sound good to you. Eat without distractions. (see distraction section)

NO | WRITE If it's not stomach hunger, what are you feeling? Jot down words/notes on your phone or in a notebook. You might not know, just brainstorm ideas.

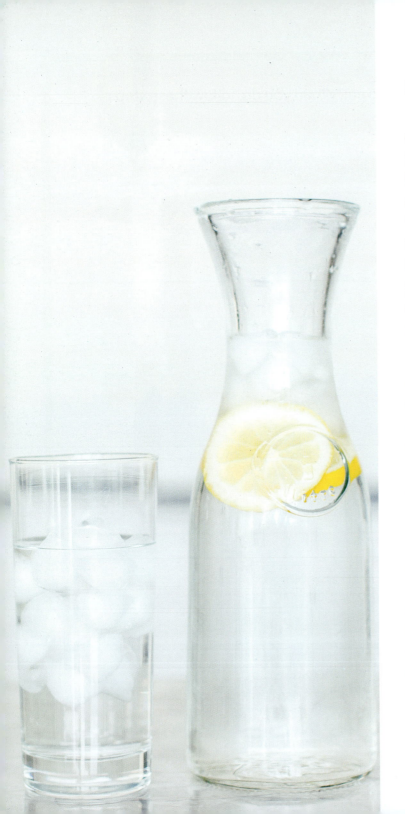

HYDRATE THE INCINERATOR

The need to drink more water is old news. Here's how it applies to your incinerator. You could easily mistake hunger for thirst, making you reach for something to eat when you are not "technically" hungry. When you are not actually physically hungry, the hormone ghrelin has not been released to signal the need for fuel. Yet, sometimes you still feel empty when you've actually had enough food. That empty feeling can be the need for fluid, not food.

Staying well hydrated will help you more clearly distinguish hunger from other feelings. Low energy or weakness, while often a sign of hunger, can also be a need for fluid. Fluid plays a strong role in detecting hunger.[45] If you're not sure whether or not you're hungry, it's highly likely you are not. You are probably just thirsty.

To explore it, drink a tall glass of water to see if the feeling disappears for a period of time. I've outlined hydration guidelines so you have an idea of how much water will keep your body and incinerator hydrated each day. This will increase your ability to decipher physical hunger from needing fluid. These are my recommendations - your baseline of water intake.

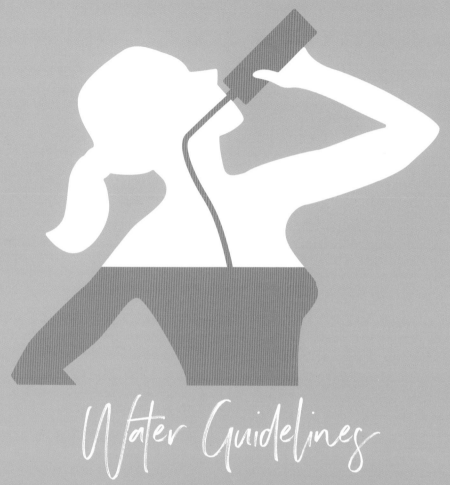

Water Guidelines

Divide your weight (lbs) in half. Those are the ounces of water you need per day to keep you well hydrated. For every hour of exercise, add 16 ounces. For example:

$$150 \text{lbs} \div 2 = 75\text{oz water per day}$$
$$+ 16\text{oz water for exercise}$$
$$91\text{oz water per day}$$

This is your general baseline of water intake per day.

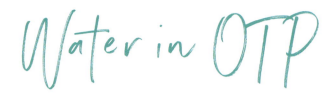

Water in OTP

- In your gut, water helps dissolve fats and soluble fiber. Adequate water helps you poop (yes, I just said that) and prevents constipation. [47] If you are regular, you feel better – you've seen the happy, regular people on commercials. That happiness is a real thing from pooping.

- Water helps you feel refreshed to the point of improving your mood.[49,50] If you feel better, you have a brighter outlook and an increased ability to keep hydrating and following ONE-TWO PUNCH.

- Water (staying hydrated) helps prevent headaches.[49,51] Who cares what you're eating or how much when you have a headache??? Many headaches are brought on by mild dehydration; easily solvable within 30 minutes of drinking 2 cups of water.[49]

- Adequate water intake helps energize you and makes you more alert[49] – more energy and more focus equal increased productivity for whatever you are trying to accomplish.

- Water keeps your joints lubricated and makes movement easier.[52] If your body is not in pain, you're going to feel better about moving.

- In the moment you realize you need water instead of food, you decrease calories by not having the food you might have eaten, thereby possibly leading to more weight loss.

For some of you it will mean significantly increasing your water intake. I'm aware that it also means you are significantly increasing the number of times you're visiting the restroom. Well, would you rather hang on to those pounds that you don't like or visit the restroom a little more often? For many, peeing more often is a small price to pay to get the benefits of drinking adequate water.

I recommend not counting soda, coffee, tea, milk, juice, sports drinks and other beverages towards your total intake of water. My experience is that people do better with a baseline of water for hydration.[25, 46-47] Treat other drinks as extra. If you hate water, you can add non-caloric flavoring such as Crystal Light™ to help you out.

REST THE INCINERATOR

Just as emotions affect your ability to sense hunger and fullness, sleep significantly influences how you behave.[35,53-55] Adequate sleep keeps you mentally sharp, reduces the stress you feel and repairs the wear and tear the body receives during it's waking hours. Inadequate sleep makes you less productive, slower in general and more stressed. The lack of sleep also weakens your immune system, making you more susceptible to illness, like a simple cold.[56]

You have less ability to access your coping skills when you are tired. So trying to figure out whether or not you're hungry gets murky. Your sleep influences your sensitivity to the hormones ghrelin and leptin and the amounts of the hormones secreted.[35,54-55,57]

Physically, with less sleep, your body tries to adapt and give you the energy you are lacking. It tries to protect itself. So what does it do? It spits out more ghrelin to make you feel hungrier and eat more. And it spits out less leptin to make you feel less full and eat more. If you are trying to lose weight, eating more is working against you.[54-55,57]

In addition to feeling hungrier, the food you crave is higher in fat and carbohydrates. With sleep deprivation, it's as if you need more bang for your buck to try to make up for lost zzzzzs. Studies have shown that after just one night of poor sleep, people craved more fatty and sugary food the next day.[35,53-55,58] All in an effort to make you feel like you have energy when what you really need is a nap!!!

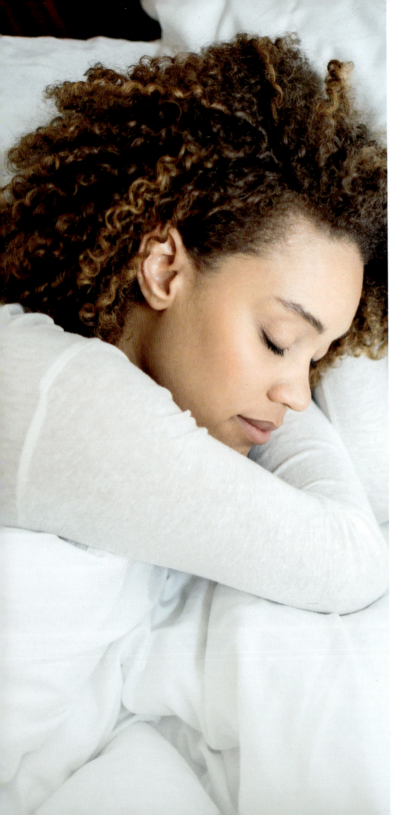

Sleep is something to be aware of when you are trying to decipher your physical sensations of hunger. You might be just plain tired. You can choose to power through with a brownie or take a rest. Obviously, resting isn't always possible. Being aware of what is happening can prompt you to do things unrelated to food to keep going.

Learning the signals of your physical hunger, with all their subtleties, will take practice. It will take practice to understand your incinerator. And it will take commitment to pay attention to the signals and all the other things that affect the system. And it will take practice to maintain the machinery. Think of it as doing maintenance checks every day.

Of course the human body and brain are much more complicated than an incinerator. For optimal health, it's important to put things into the incinerator in a particular way. Let's move on to discover how nutrients should be combined as you put them into your body.

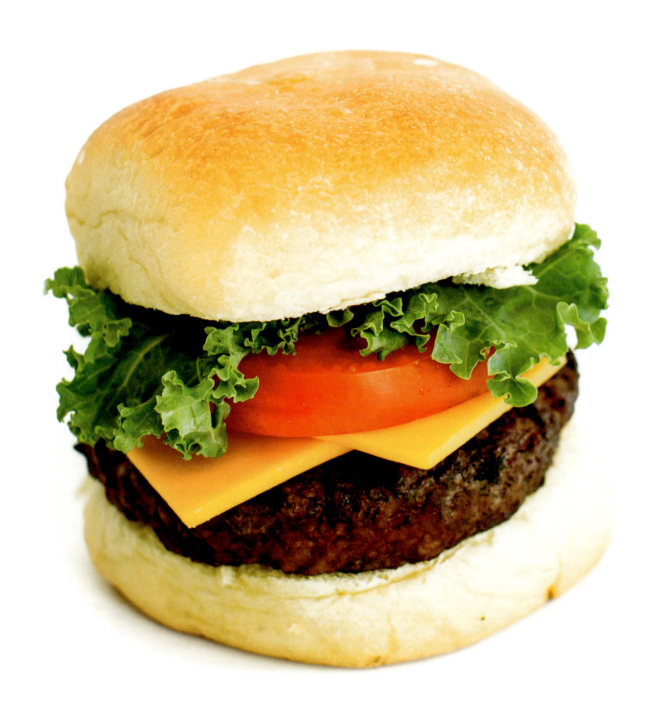

BALANCE

The first foundational principle, BURN, might be the hardest of all — to distinguish physical hunger. The principle of BALANCE is designed to help you regulate and stabilize your physical hunger and fullness. We do this by balancing the carbohydrate and protein entering your stomach (incinerator) and then your bloodstream.

THE PROTEIN ANCHOR

When you eat a carbohydrate by itself, without any protein and/or fat, it enters your body in a particular way. Those carbs hit your bloodstream, spike your blood sugar and exit just as quickly.[59-60] Let's say you followed the first principle of BURN and ate those carbs when you were hungry. Your hunger might temporarily vanish, but you'll be hungry again soon, even though you might have "theoretically" had enough calories to keep you full. That's because the carbs swam into the bloodstream without an anchor slowing them down. Being slowed down in this sense is a good thing so you feel full longer.

For example, imagine you are hungry and you decide to have a concession-size box of Red Vine™ Licorice, which doesn't have any fat or protein. Those carbs would enter your bloodstream, spike your blood sugar and leave the bloodstream about as quickly, leaving you hungry again.[59,61] Instead, consider half a bagel with a full-fat shmear of cream cheese along with some turkey. That would enter your bloodstream more slowly,

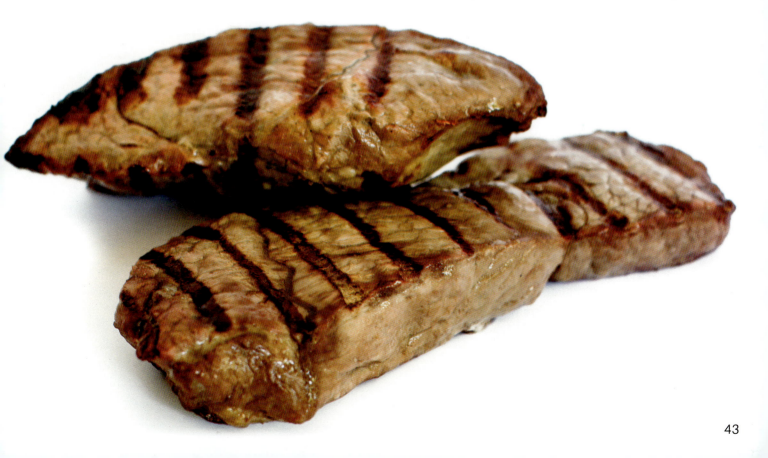

stay longer and exit more slowly.[60-63] You would be full, for fewer calories, for a longer period of time. It's difficult to feel full when eating carbohydrates alone.[59,64-65]

So, you've had a lot of calories without making you feel particularly full. Carbs eaten alone prompt a particular insulin response to take care of the sugar rush and its effects on your blood sugar. Insulin is a hormone that works to move glucose from your blood and distribute it to other parts of your body.

It is released every time you eat and the more carbohydrate you eat, the more insulin you need to take care of the rise in blood sugar. Eating protein or fat alone does not raise blood sugar significantly enough to require an insulin response. Adding protein or fat to a carbohydrate food can change how the insulin responds to that food as it enters the blood stream. Lowering the amount of carbohydrate food you eat will require less insulin to be released. Combining a carbohydrate food with protein and/or fat will modify your insulin response.

If you are eating carbohydrates frequently throughout the day, unaccompanied by any protein and/or fat, you've also got a lot of insulin being secreted in your body again and again.[61]

Insulin distributes glucose throughout your body for use, but is also a hormone that promotes fat storage. When all the glucose needs of the body are met, the leftover glucose is converted into fat storage.[66] When you have a lot of insulin floating around your bloodstream and body, there is more potential to have increased fat storage and to feel hungry more often.[40] This happens when you eat more carbs, or food in general, than the body can use. In ONE-TWO PUNCH we want to manage your insulin response and help you feel full longer, thus secreting less insulin.[60,62]

This concept is worth repeating again in a different way. When you eat a carbohydrate ALONE, without protein or fat, blood sugar can rise quickly. Without anything to slow it down, like protein or fat, your blood sugar can "spike" and then be followed by a significant drop. With low blood sugar, your body will probably respond with hunger or need a "pick-me-up" and you naturally reach for more carbohydrates, the preferred fuel source.[66] Without anchoring the carbohydrate, you are hungry more often.[67]

When you eat a carbohydrate combined with a protein source, its entrance into the bloodstream is slowed down, thus

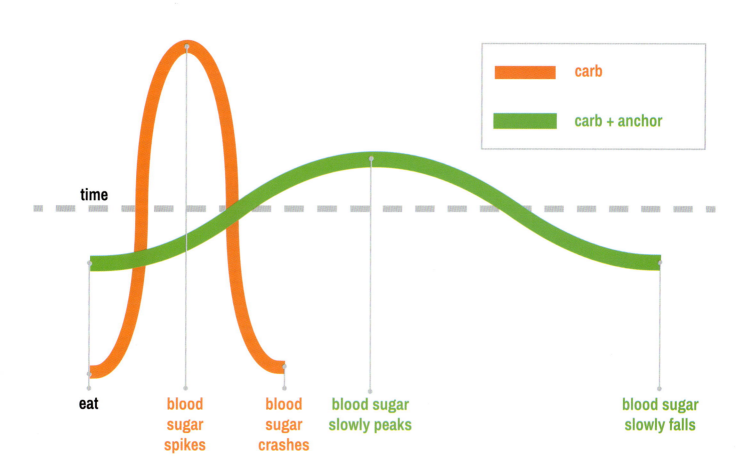

stabilizing blood sugar: the rise is slower, it stays longer and there's not a severe drop after the spike.[59] This has several advantages. Because protein serves as a blood sugar stabilizer, you don't repeatedly get hungry and continue to reach for more carbohydrates.

The more you reach for carbohydrates, the more calories you consume and the more insulin you need to help clear sugar from the blood. The more insulin released, the more potential there is to store fat. Are you seeing a pattern here?

In addition, protein helps maintain fullness.[60,62-63,68] One of the challenges of dieting is getting hungry. Feeling full longer can be of great benefit when trying to lose weight. If you have a protein with that carbohydrate, you will likely consume fewer calories and stay full, or at least satisfied, for a few hours.

Adding protein or fat slows the carbohydrate down as it enters your bloodstream.[59,69-70] Protein and fat serve as anchors in your bloodstream, preventing the carbohydrate from peaking too fast. Your insulin responds differently too, based on the combination of nutrients entering your bloodstream.[59] It is valuable to ALWAYS have a carbohydrate with a protein, and not have a carbohydrate food by itself.

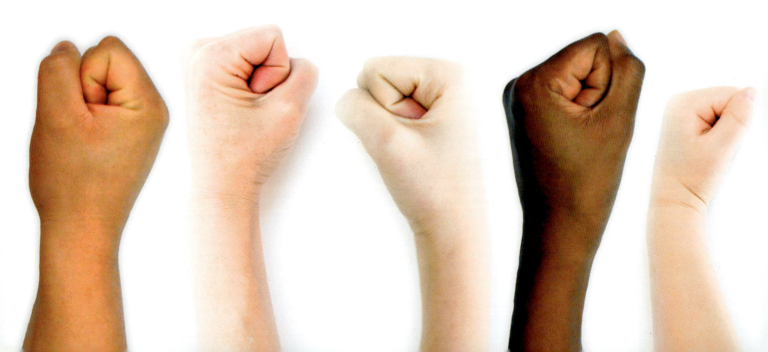

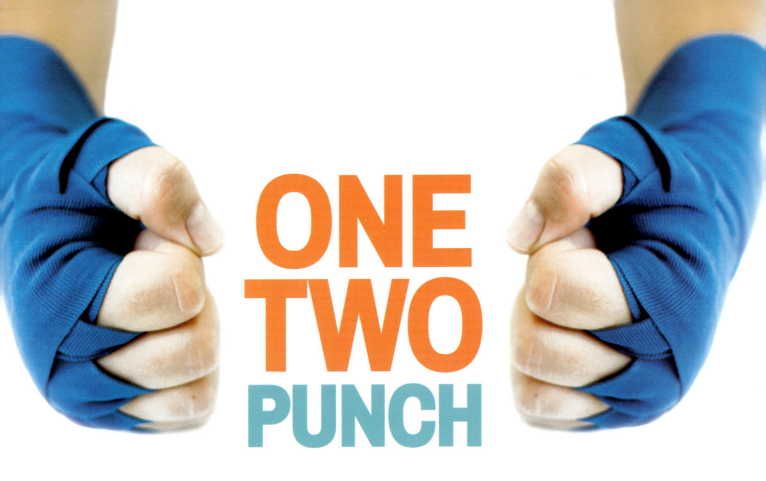

ONE TWO PUNCH

Eating a fist-size serving of carbs with a fist-size serving of protein creates the perfect "ONE-TWO PUNCH." Carbs alone are digested very quickly causing a spike, followed by a drop in blood sugar, leaving you feeling hungry faster.

Pairing carbs with a protein slows the digestion of carbs and balances the blood sugar levels. This keeps you satisfied longer.

ONE-TWO PUNCH

Remember I told you this book would teach you to eat in a balanced way without measuring, tracking, weighing or calculating? Make a fist; that's the portion size of carbohydrate and the portion size of protein you need EVERY time you're hungry and decide to eat. The size of your fists represents your ONE-TWO PUNCH, your knockout combo, a fist of carb and a fist of protein.[71] There it is!

The beauty of the "fist and fist" method is that it's not MY fist size, it's yours. You should see the relief on some clients' faces when I say that! My clients that are male, over six feet tall and around 250 pounds are very relieved to learn it's not the size of MY fist and that they're not going to starve! It's the size of your own individual, unique fist. This is the magical part of ONE-TWO PUNCH that works for ANY age, 2 years old to 97 years old. It's easy to determine serving and portion sizes, ANYWHERE, ANY TIME, at ANY AGE with the size of your fists.

Why the fist? Because you need something tangible, but you need it without the stress of measurement. If all of us knew how to eat in moderation, everyone would already be doing it. But eating in moderation is too variable, too subjective and too abstract.[72] It doesn't take into account the texture, volume, density and color of the food and doesn't account for plate size and other factors.

The fists help you with portion control while you learn to eat for hunger and satisfaction. Think of them as training wheels or a safety net for your practice of eating mindfully.

I get a lot of questions about the dimensions of the fist. You want to think of it more like a box; a 3-dimensional object more than a 2-dimensional outline. For example, if you were to roughly smash a piece of bread up into a ball, would it be the size of your fist or only half that size? We're looking for the total volume of your fist: one fist of carb and one fist of protein.

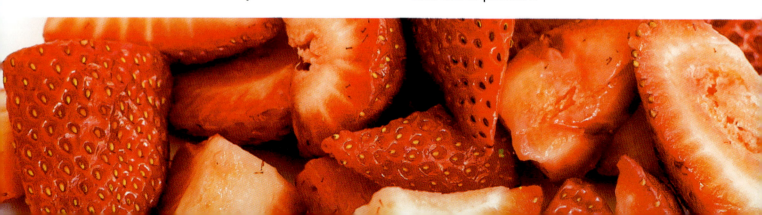

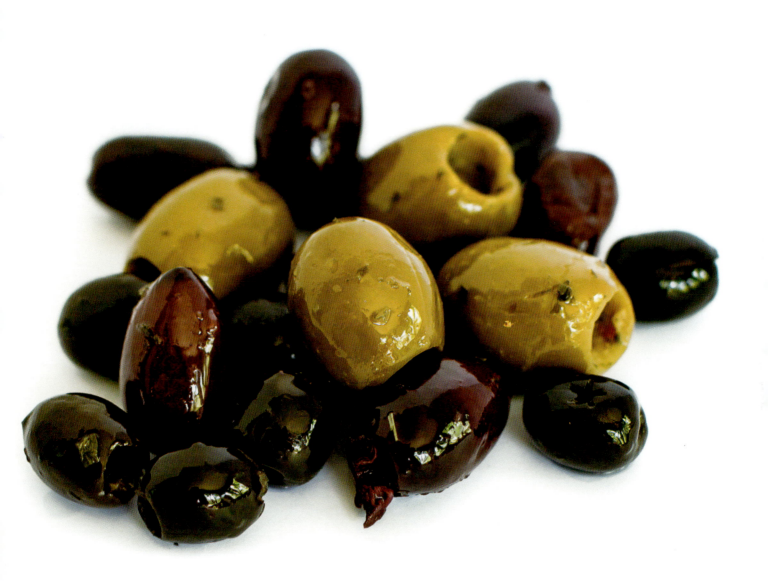

This could be you!

For starters, I have never had a weight problem, but I have had a carb problem. I have always been somewhat active and have tried to be aware of what I was eating. I have never been one to diet because restricting myself always backfires.

The stress of a bad marriage, and basically being a single parent, took a toll on my ability to be aware of what I was eating. Cooking is not my thing, so I was eating whatever food was in the pantry or eating out all the time. Neither of these things led to making good food choices. I realized I was eating a TON of processed carbs and sugar in between meals and I was not eating anything of substance for dinner.

Eventually, after a divorce, I was able to focus on me. I was able to implement a good fitness routine that provided physical pain relief. But, I was sabotaging my fitness efforts with ice cream, cookies and candy. I realized it was time for me to make a meaningful change in my eating habits. Unfortunately, I had forgotten how to eat healthy and I knew that removing the stuff I love to eat (carbs) would not be helpful. Life has carbs whether you like it or not.

I found ONE-TWO PUNCH on Instagram. I thought, "I like this idea of balancing my carbs with a protein and this seems easy to understand and put into practice." I also knew that portion control is a weakness for me. I am 5'9" and muscular so eating tiny portions leaves me hungry which leads me to overeat. Of course I was hungry because I was eating processed carbs without substance and not nearly enough protein. My idea of a healthy dinner was noodles with tons of veggies. Learning about OTP led me to realize that by not balancing my carbs with a protein I was just constantly yearning for more food.

Through OTP I have realized that I can have my once weekly donut if I add a strong protein like eggs. My meals have more stamina and don't leave me grazing on goldfish and ice cream. I now try to keep sources of protein on hand. I like that OTP doesn't preach "fat-free" foods and no butter or oil, but instead includes fat to help fill me up.

I need eating healthy to be easy, not overly complicated and not expensive. ONE-TWO PUNCH allows me to tailor it to my likes and wants. I see my tastes turning away from highly processed carbs and moving more towards carbs with substance. In the end it is all about balance. Thank you for promoting a method based on common sense and balance. Thank you for promoting a method that doesn't take all the flavor and fun out of eating.

-Abby

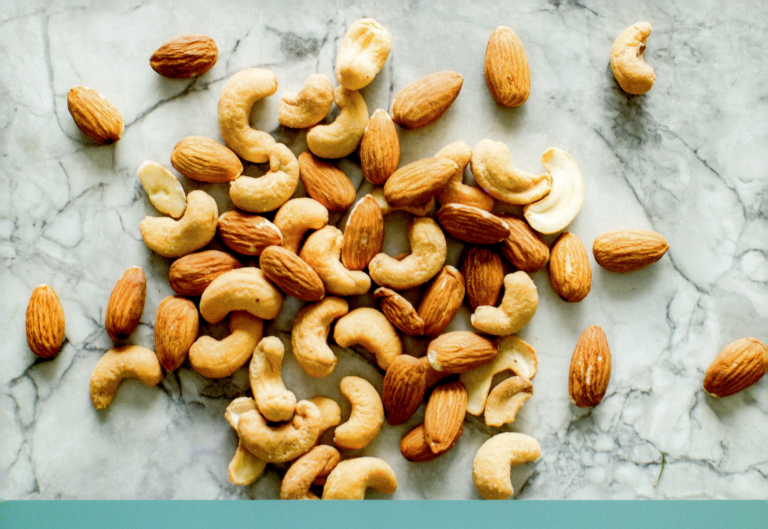

NUT CHART

	ALMOND	BRAZIL	CASHEW	HAZELNUT	MACADAMIA	PECAN	PISTACHIO	WALNUT
PROTEIN	6	4.1	5.2	4.2	2.2	2.6	5.8	4.3
CARBS	6.1	3.5	8.6	4.7	3.9	3.9	7.8	3.9
FAT	14	18.8	12.4	17.2	21.5	20.4	12.9	18.5

grams per 1/2 cup

Carbohydrates include foods such as fruit (yes, fruit), fruit juices, bread, cereal, crackers, grains, rice, pasta, candy, regular sugar soda, cake, cookies, pies, ice cream and starchy vegetables like potatoes, corn and peas.[73]

Technically, non-starchy vegetables are a carbohydrate. However, they do not contribute enough carbohydrates to include them as a carb. These include vegetables such as lettuce, cucumbers, broccoli, cauliflower, green beans and others.

Proteins include foods such as meats, eggs, cheese, Greek yogurt, nuts, nut butters, tofu, protein powders and other plant-based proteins.[74]

While nuts are considered by some nutritionists to be fats, in ONE-TWO PUNCH they are considered protein. Yes, most of the calories in nuts come from fat, roughly 80 percent. But they also contain about 14 percent protein and 6 percent carbohydrate.

A standard serving of nuts contains about as much protein as one egg, one ounce of meat or a cheese stick. For most people, a fist of nuts is roughly two servings, meaning you are getting the protein equivalent of two eggs, 2 ounces of meat or two cheese sticks.

I know that's a lot of calories and a lot of fat. I know. But if you're following the first foundational principle of OTP and eating when you're hungry, the fat in the nuts or nut butter is going to keep you full for a very long time, so you won't be eating as often.

I think of the fat in nuts and nut butters as boosting the overall anchoring effect of the food. A protein food with fat is more anchoring to your carbohydrate. For example, a grilled chicken breast has lots of protein, but will have more staying power if a fat is also added, like dressing on a salad. Nuts and nut butters have the anchoring boost of fat built in.

In ONE-TWO PUNCH, fat is treated as a condiment that will add to your feelings of fullness and satisfaction.[75] If you're using the fist as your parameter, you can keep the fat intake in check. Yes, nuts are super tasty, and it would be easy to go overboard and eat a container of cashews. But you're using your fist as your portion guide.

In ONE-TWO PUNCH, fat is not included as a macronutrient you need to count in your fists of protein and carbohydrate. It is considered a condiment; butter on your vegetables, dressing on your salad or fat already in your choice of protein or

Take it just one step, one meal, at a time.

carbohydrate. Fats include oils, cream, butter, margarine, salad dressing, avocados and some sauces.

There is fat in some of the carbohydrate and protein foods that you choose as your fist-sized portions, but the idea is not to get too caught up in the details. Remember, if you're using your fists as your portion guidelines, your fat is not going to be out of control. Some meals will be higher in fat than others. With more fat in some meals you will stay full for a longer period of time. Remember the first foundational principle is waiting until you are hungry before eating.

So you've got foods designated as protein, foods designated as carbohydrate and fat as a condiment. However, not every food fits neatly into a category. Some foods contain a mixture of nutrients; some naturally contain protein and carbohydrates and some have a mixture of both because of the way they are prepared.

Food prepared with both carbohydrate and protein, by putting two different foods together, are considered mixed foods in ONE-TWO PUNCH. These include foods such as lasagna, casseroles, macaroni and cheese, pizza and so on.

Foods that already have protein and carbohydrate in them naturally are considered a hybrid food in ONE-TWO PUNCH. The protein and carb is contained in one food. Such is the case with legumes because they contain a combination of both carbohydrate and protein.

For example, a half-cup of black beans contains 7-8 grams of protein and 20+ grams of carbohydrate. That's as much protein as a cheese stick but they're lopsided a bit towards carbs. And while they contain about 15 grams fiber that contributes to fullness, they don't have the staying power that fats provide, like in nuts. Due to the protein, legumes don't fit completely into the carbohydrate category. In ONE-TWO PUNCH legumes are a hybrid food.

Here's how a hybrid food works in OTP. If you're having hummus, one fist-size serving would contain a half-fist of protein and a half-fist of carb. That's what I mean by hybrid. Have two fistfuls of hummus with fresh cut-up veggies. You're already getting your carb. You're already getting your protein. Having two fistfuls is like having a fist of each.

If you have the hummus with pita bread or chips, your carb intake becomes lopsided and out of balance. If you're having a

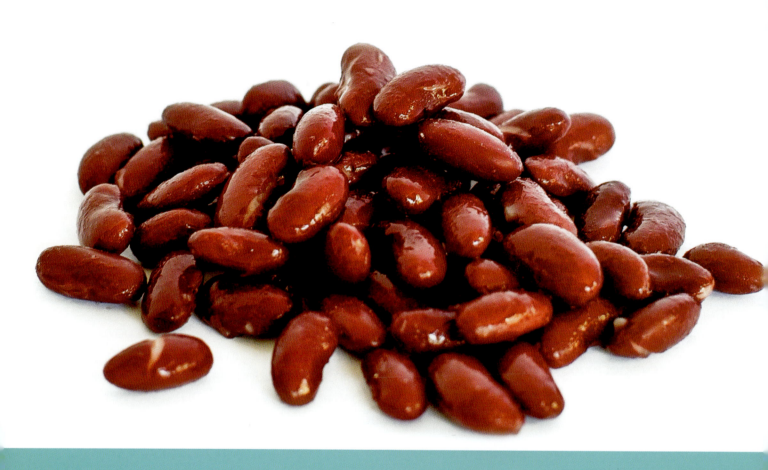

LEGUME CHART

	BLACK BEANS	GARBANZO BEANS	KIDNEY BEANS	LENTILS	NAVY BEANS	PINTO BEANS	SPLIT PEAS
PROTEIN	8	6	8	9	8	8	9
CARBS	20	27	20	20	24	22	21
FAT	.5	2	.4	0	.6	.6	0

grams per 1/2 cup

small cup of lentil soup, it's both protein and carbohydrate. If you add a piece of bread, that's more carb. You're going to be sustained longer and feel more satisfied if you also add some protein to the bread and soup. Or have a larger bowl of soup because it already contains both.

I am aware that many vegans and vegetarians use legumes solely as a protein, for instance with rice. This idea came from obtaining particular amino acids from the legumes and different amino acids from the rice to make a complete protein. Specifics regarding amino acids are outside the scope of this book. Our focus is the protein and carbohydrate available from food and how it enters the body. Legumes have more carbohydrate than protein but still have both components in one food. They are considered a hybrid food in ONE-TWO PUNCH.

Milk is also considered a hybrid food in OTP. It used to be that when someone said milk, everyone knew they were talking about cow milk – that was the only available option. Now, there's rice milk, almond milk, hemp

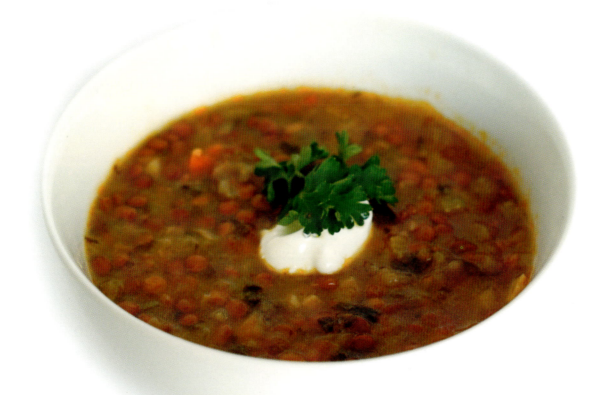

MILK CHART

	PROTEIN	CARBS	FATS
SKIM MILK	8	13	0
1% MILK	8	13	2.5
2% MILK	8	12	3.5
WHOLE MILK	8	12	8
PLAIN ALMOND MILK, UNSWEETENED	1	0	2.5
VANILLA ALMOND MILK	1	16	2.5
PLAIN CASHEW MILK, UNSWEETENED	0	1	2
VANILLA CASHEW MILK	0	14	2.5
PLAIN COCONUT MILK, UNSWEETENED	0	0	4.5
VANILLA COCONUT MILK	0	10	5
PLAIN HEMP MILK, UNSWEETENED	3	1	5
VANILLA HEMP MILK	3	24	5
PLAIN RICE MILK, UNSWEETENED	0	15	2.5
VANILLA RICE MILK	1	26	2.5
UNSWEETENED SOY MILK	7	4	4
VANILLA SOY MILK	6	10	3.5

grams per 1 cup

milk, flaxseed milk, coconut milk, soy milk, goat milk, oat milk and more. And within each of these types there are subtypes — sweetened, unsweetened, vanilla flavored, non-fat, reduced-fat and full-fat. So many choices!!!

I'm going to use cow milk as an example for starters and explain how it fits into ONE-TWO PUNCH. A cup of cow milk has 8 grams of protein, about the same as a cheese stick. It also has around 13 grams of carbs, near the carbs in a slice of bread. So, consider a glass of cow milk a hybrid food — it has both carbohydrate and protein.

It's the same for a cup of regular, not Greek, plain cow milk yogurt. It's a hybrid food and that's just the plain version! When you add fruit and/or sugar, you're adding another carb and it's like you've got two fists of carbs to one fist protein. With Greek yogurt, much of the lactose or milk sugar is strained out. It then becomes higher in protein and lower in carbohydrate. That's why OTP considers plain Greek yogurt a protein. When Greek yogurt has fruit and/or sugar included, it's already a balance of a fist of carb and a fist of protein.

So how should you treat all the other milks in ONE-TWO PUNCH? I hesitate laying down guidelines, as I don't want you to get caught up in the details that will cause this to unravel. Remember, we are into simple – waaaay into simple. But I also understand you need some parameters.

Here they are:

If a milk has around 8 grams of protein and less than 5 grams of carbohydrate, it serves as a protein. If a milk has more than 10 grams of carbs, it should be considered a carbohydrate serving. It can also serve as a protein serving if it meets the requirement of around 8 grams of protein. What if a serving of milk has 4 grams of protein and about 6 grams of carbohydrate? It doesn't pack enough punch to be considered as a significant source of either protein or carbohydrate. Go ahead and use it, but use it in addition to your fist of protein and fist of carbohydrate. This might be over cereal, in smoothies and in recipes. In this case, the

> **Remember, we are into simple – waaaay into simple.**

milk serves as a condiment in much the same way that fat does.

The last few pages include a lot of chatter and graphs about grams of carbohydrate, protein and fat. I included this for factual information, comparison and example. It would be easy to go down the rabbit hole with the particular grams of carbohydrate, protein and fat of various food items. You'll drive yourself crazy trying to categorize every single food.

To stabilize your blood sugar and prolong fullness, the fist of carbohydrate and fist of protein do not need to be gram for gram. A 2:1 ratio of carbohydrate to protein will still be effective. For example, a piece of bread has roughly 15-20 grams carbohydrate. Depending on the size of your fist, this could be your fist-size portion of carbohydrate. A cheese stick has about 8 grams of protein. This could be your other fist. Or, you might need two cheese sticks. A fist-size portion of chicken breast might have 3 times the amount of protein. That exact ratio of carbohydrate to protein will change based on the food items you choose.

The important component of the BALANCE principle is to include an estimated fist-sized portion of protein to accompany the carbs you are eating, every time you eat. Do the best you can in choosing items that are appealing to you and then remember the principle of BURN – what still matters is eating when you're hungry.

A WORD ABOUT ALCOHOL

Technically, alcohol is a different nutrient than a carbohydrate, protein or fat. For the purpose of ONE-TWO PUNCH, especially if trying to lose weight, a serving of alcohol (beer, wine, whiskey, liqueur) is considered a carbohydrate. If you are trying to lose weight and you really want a beer with your burger, you might want to choose a lettuce wrap burger as your protein and choose the beer as your carbohydrate.

> If you really want a beer with your burger, you might want to choose a lettuce wrap burger as your protein and choose the beer as your carbohydrate.

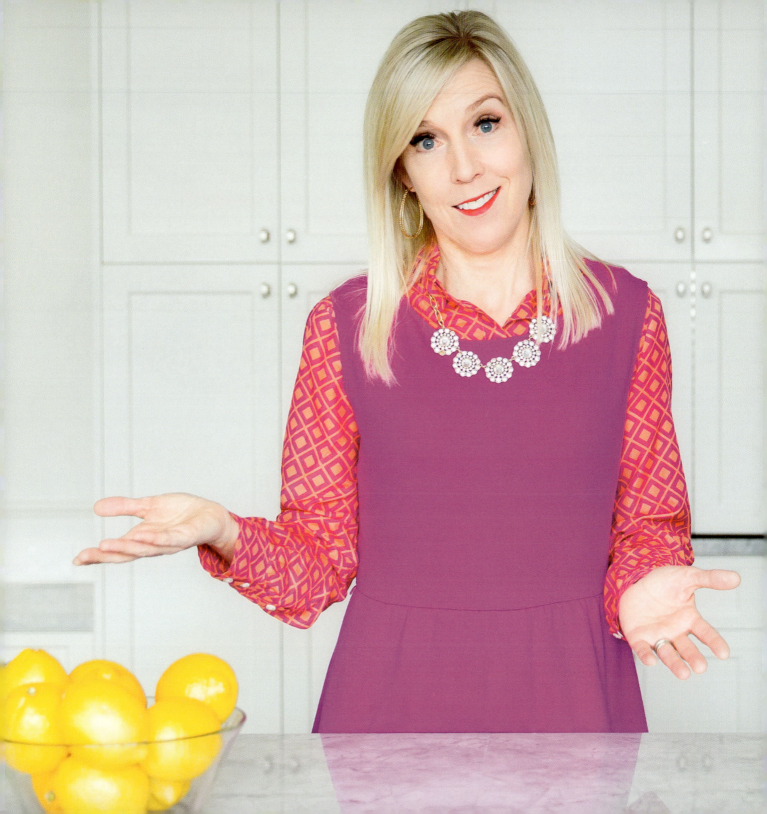

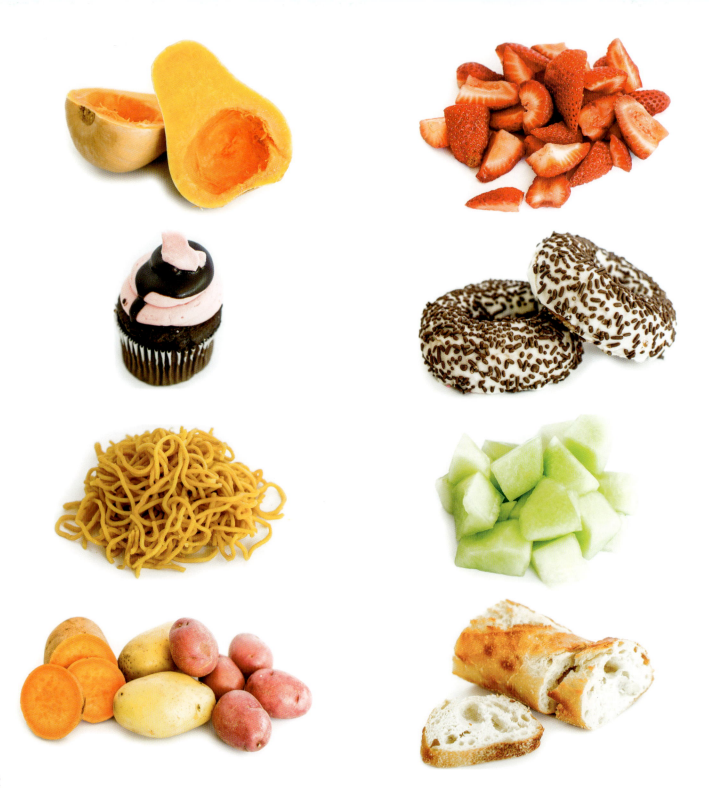

Carbohydrates are the body's main source of energy and are required for proper function of the brain, central nervous system and kidneys.

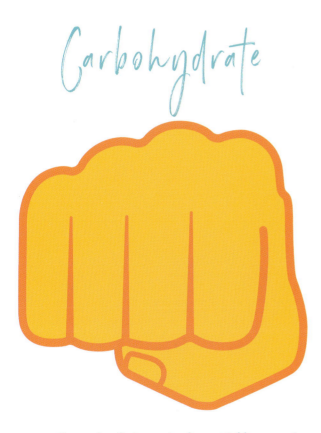

Carbohydrate

Remember that non-starchy vegetables are not counted as carbohydrates.

Fresh Fruit
apple
applesauce
apricot
banana
blackberries
blueberries
cantaloupe
cherries
figs
grapefruit
grapes
honeydew
kiwi
mango
nectarine
orange
peach
pear
pineapple
plum
raspberries
strawberries
watermelon

Fruit Juice
apple juice
cranberry juice
orange juice
pineapple juice
prune juice
fruit juice blends

Vegetables
potato
sweet potato
yam
pumpkin
corn
peas
winter squash

Grains
pasta
brown rice
hamburger buns
bread
roll
bagel
English muffin
crackers
pancake
pita bread
tortilla
frozen waffles

Cereal
oatmeal
grits
bran flakes
granola
cereal (sweetened/unsweetened)
shredded wheat
bulgur
wheat germ

Crackers/Snacks
popcorn
pretzels
animal crackers
graham crackers
club crackers
oyster crackers
saltine crackers
potato chips
tortilla chips
rice cakes

Desserts/Pastries
angel food cake
eclair
danish
brownie
cake
cookies
doughnut
pie
sweet roll
ice cream
sherbert/sorbet
frozen yogurt
candy
chocolate
caramel

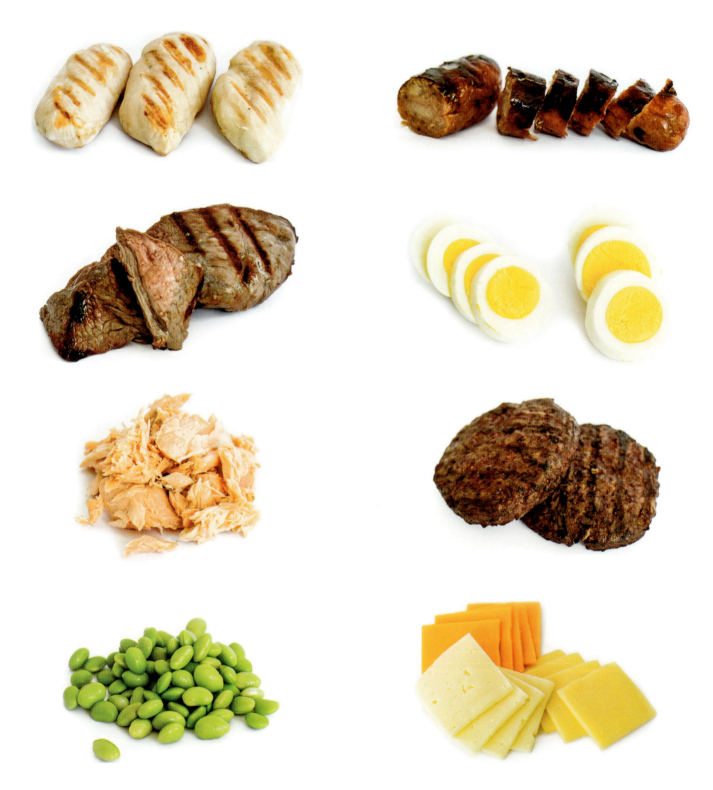

Proteins are used by the body for tissue repair, muscle maintenance, growth and the production of hormones and enzymes.

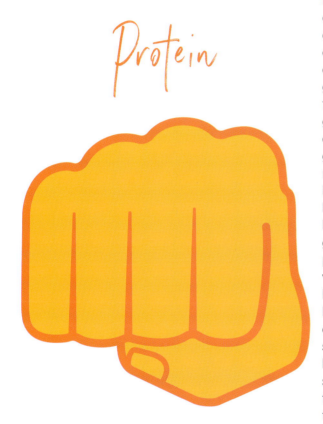

Protein

Meat
chicken breast
chicken leg
chicken wing
chicken thigh
ground chicken
turkey breast
ground turkey
duck
goose
rabbit
lamb chop
lamb ribs
lamb roast
ground lamb
pheasant
venison
buffalo
bison
oysters
sardines
halibut
salmon
tilapia
tuna
trout
crab
lobster
shrimp
veal
corned beef
short ribs
prime rib
top sirloin steak
flank steak
beef tenderloin
beef ribs
beef roast
porter house steak
cubed beef
ground beef
Canadian bacon
pork tenderloin
pork chop
pork cutlets
pork butt
lean ham
hot dog
kidney
sausage
jerky
deli meat

Dairy
cottage cheese
hard cheese
Mozzarella
Feta
Ricotta
Parmesan
plain Greek yogurt

Alternatives
tofu
textured vegetable
 protein (tvp)
tempeh
seitan
veggie burger
eggs
egg substitute
whey protein
 powder
hemp protein
 powder
plant based protein
 powder
edamame
soymilk

Nuts/Seeds
peanut butter
almond butter
cashew butter
almonds
cashews
peanuts
hazelnuts
madamia nuts
pecans
pumpkin seeds
sunflower seeds
sesame seeds

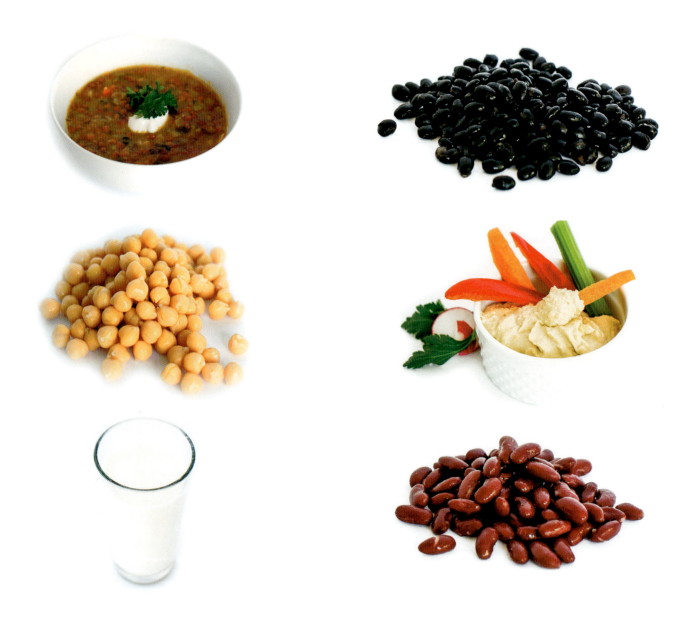

Hybrid foods have both protein and carbohydrates. They include legumes, beans and dairy (except for cheese).

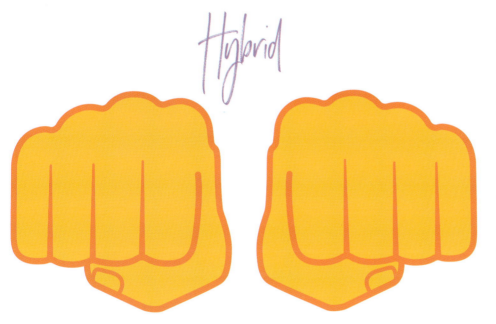

Legumes
black beans
baked beans
cannellini beans
navy beans
kidney beans
fava beans
lima beans
pinto beans
lentils
chickpeas
split peas
hummus

Dairy
milk
plain yogurt
buttermilk

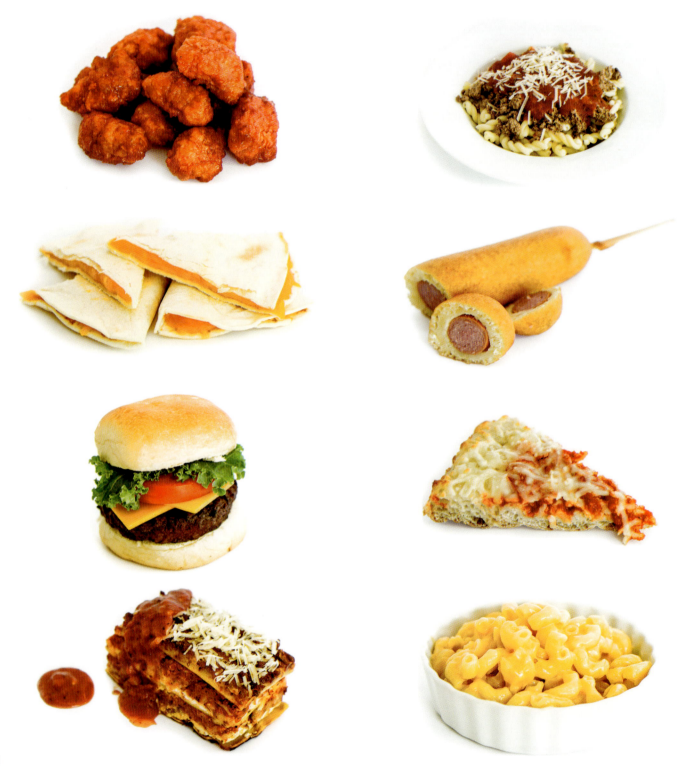

Mixed foods are two different foods combined together to offer a carbohydrate and protein in one entree.

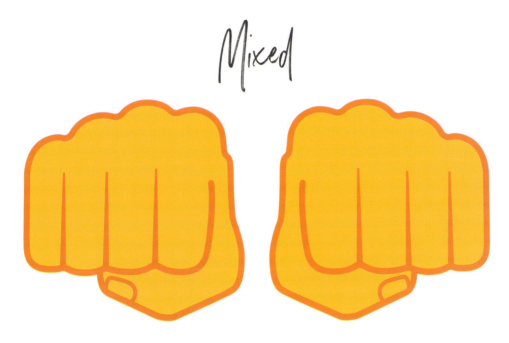

Mixed

Pizza/Pasta
cheese pizza
pepperoni pizza
meat pizza
macaroni and cheese
lasagna
baked ziti
spaghetti & meatballs
cheese ravioli

Soup
bean
chicken noodle
beef vegetables

One Pot Dinners
casseroles
hot dishes
chicken & dumplings
goulash
beef stroganoff

Sandwiches
hamburger
sloppy joes
hot ham & cheese
grilled cheese
cheesesteak
meatball sandwich

Other
corndog
sushi rolls
quesadilla
orange chicken

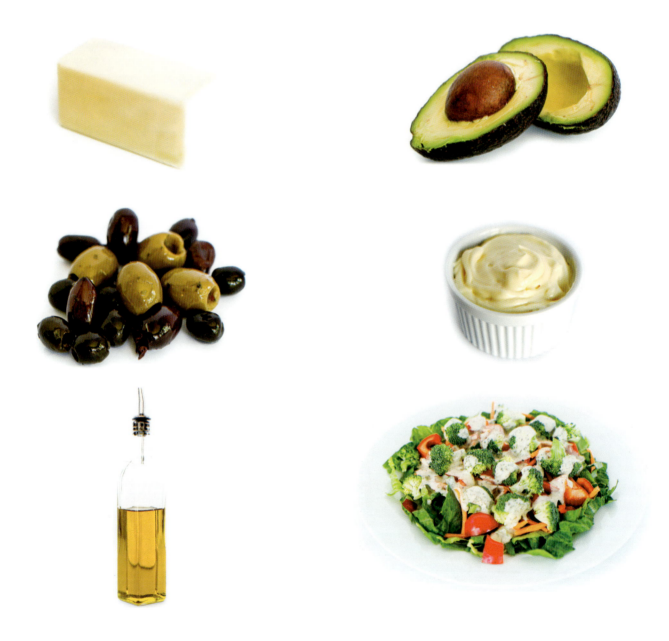

Fats are used in the maintenace of cell membranes, help cushion organs and provide insulation for the body. Fats are also an energy source.

Oil
canola oil
coconut oil
olive oil
vegetable oil
flaxseed oil
avocado oil
grapeseed oil
corn oil
soybean oil
safflower oil
peanut oil

Dairy
butter
sour cream
cream
half & half
heavy cream
whipping cream

Fruit
avocado
olives
coconut

Animal
salt pork
shortening
lard

Dressings/Condiments
margarine
mayonaise
Miracle Whip
salad dressing

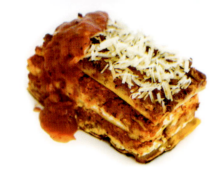
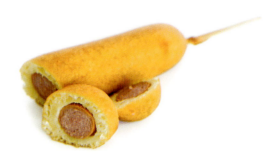
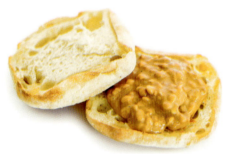
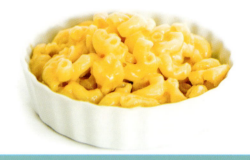

Protein + Carb Combos

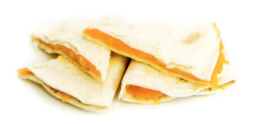
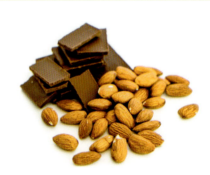
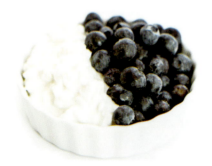
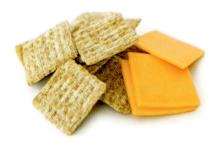

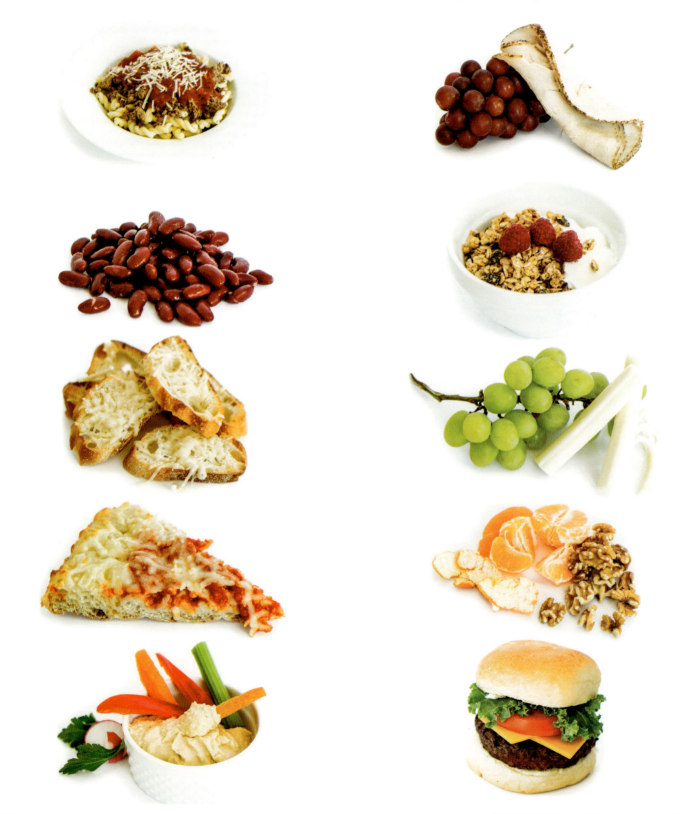

PORTION DISTORTION

ONE-TWO PUNCH allows you to get serious about portion control.[71] Sometimes, when you follow a diet, you're focusing on *what* you eat, by cutting out food groups and not *how much* you eat. It's important that you view foods a little more equally and lose the judgment. With this shift you are less likely to demonize some foods as bad and overeat foods you view as good.

OTP can be viewed as a method of portion control, sure. But portion control sounds boring and can be viewed as stressful. When I think of portion control I think of measuring, which is what you are trying to avoid. There are many factors that affect how much you eat – how it looks, smells, tastes, but also the portion you're served and the protion in relation to the plate, bowl or the size of the container.[12]

There's a tendency to think that the amount of food you're served is the amount you should eat. None of these factors take into account your body size, your metabolic needs or how hungry you are!!! Sure, weighing and measuring food portions is an accurate reflection of what is in a food. But measuring is not always practical or fun and it can be stressful.

ONE-TWO PUNCH is trying to eliminate the need to worry about body size, metabolic needs, nutrient balance, number of calories and blah, blah, blah. Your fist and fist in OTP simplifies things for you.

Plus, by using your fists as your guide, you will be immune to the ever increasing portion sizes with the accompanying plate or container sizes. And your fists are portable. You can portion control anywhere!

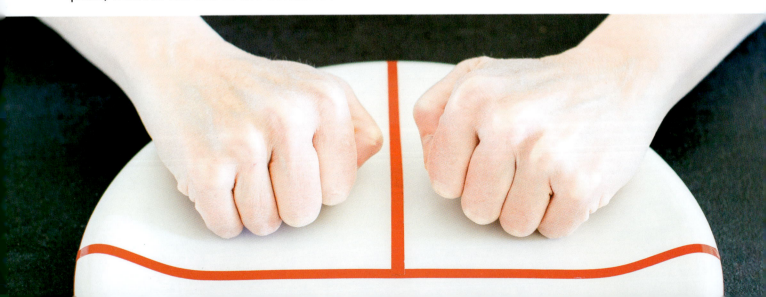

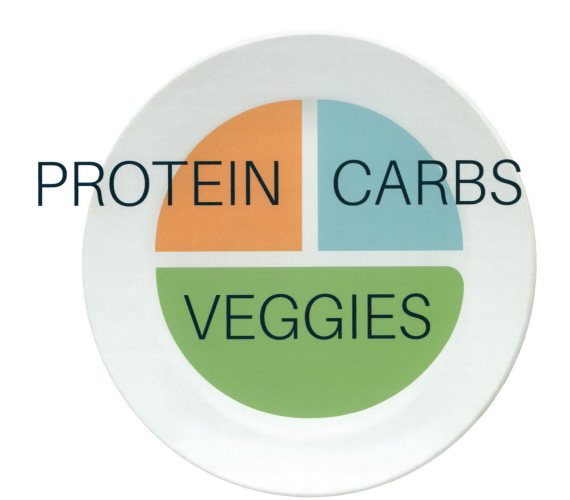
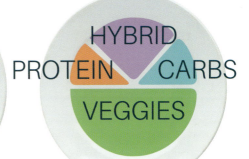

Another way to think of your portions is to visualize a plate in fractions. This should be done at each meal AND snack.

PERMISSION

Permission is a very important part of ONE-TWO PUNCH. The fist of protein can be ANY protein and the fist of carb can be ANY carbohydrate. ANY. Let's pretend this book began by telling you that in order to be healthy, all you have to do is stop having any form of sugar — cut it out entirely.

As you are trying to read this book, cutting out sugar would be invading every sentence you read. You might be reading about hydration, but all you can think about is the sugar you have to cut out to be healthy.

Or think about the last time you went on a defined, regimented diet. There's some excitement about trying something bright, shiny and new with all its promise, but also some nagging dread about all the things you cannot have. Eventually, the dread sets in and takes over anything that was exciting. Before long the dread is all you can think about; everything that's not allowed on a diet. It represents an all-or-nothing mentality, which is oozing with opportunities to fail and feel deprived.

When I meet with clients in my office I say this, "For the next 5 minutes, don't look at my earrings." Most eyes go STRAIGHT to the earrings. They didn't even notice my earrings ... *until I said that*. Suddenly, there's interest in my earrings. It's the same with ANYTHING you're told to cut out of your diet. All you can think about is the thing you're not allowed to eat. In this situation, the thing you've cut out has too much control.

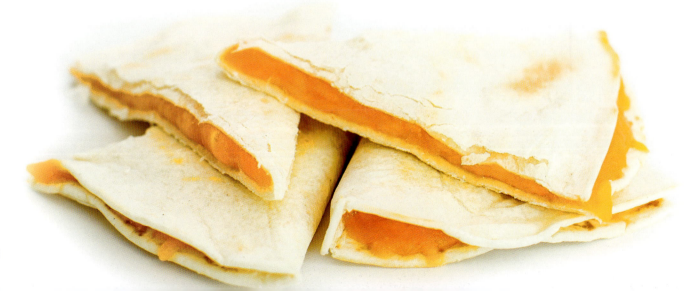

AN ALL OR NOTHING MENTALITY IS OOZING WITH OPPORTUNITIES TO FAIL

Find balance.

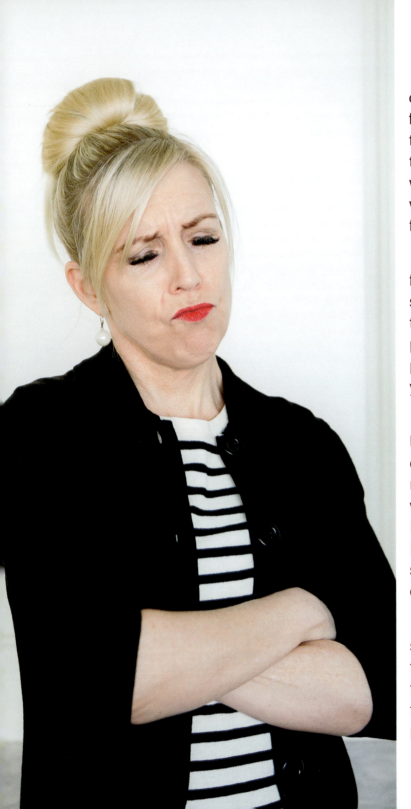

When you label certain foods as bad and off limits, they become the elusive, forbidden fruit and therefore more alluring. This gives those foods more power, making you crave them more than you typically would.[14] Then, when you eat that food, you feel guilty, which becomes another emotional trigger for overeating.

I call this the power dynamic. When you feel you can't have something, that particular something has all the power. Remember that food will not harm you as long as you practice moderation. We want to upset that power balance and give the power back to you!

While we're talking about permission, let's talk about the "cheat day." I think the entire notion of a cheat day is hysterical. I mean, think about what we're saying. Are we actually building in a day to be immoral? Dishonest? Isn't that what cheating is? I get that you want to feel rewarded by strictly adhering to a plan, but rewarded by cheating?

Okay, I'll stop asking questions. I'm just saying it sounds really backward when you think about it. Cheating implies that you've taken a very wrong turn and it also implies that you should feel guilty. If you keep portions in check, regardless of what you eat, there won't be a need to cheat or feel guilty.

Without permission, you're left with guilt about the food you ate; that you weren't "allowed" or supposed to eat. For some people the guilt becomes overwhelming. Guilt can lead to feelings of bitterness, anger, defensiveness, isolation and helplessness. These feelings can then lead to low self-esteem and the accompanying negative and unhelpful feelings about yourself.[76-77]

With all this going on, it's easy to feel defeated in your quest to become more healthy.[14] All because you feel guilty over eating a certain food? Really? Ironically, people frequently end up overeating to comfort themselves about the guilt, aka throwing in the towel.[77-78] It's easy to use food to escape or numb the feelings of guilt — even when the guilt was over food in the first place. This is a useless round and round activity, a downward spiral that only gives short-term relief.

Your reaction to guilt can drain you mentally, emotionally and physically, leaving you lacking the energy you need to take action in a positive direction. When you are tired and feeling drained, it is difficult to feel positive about anything! It's no wonder so many people eventually go off an all-or-nothing, strict diet plan. They just can't take it anymore and with good reason.

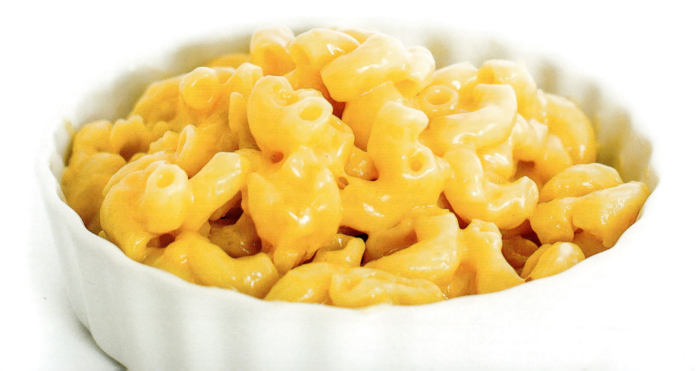

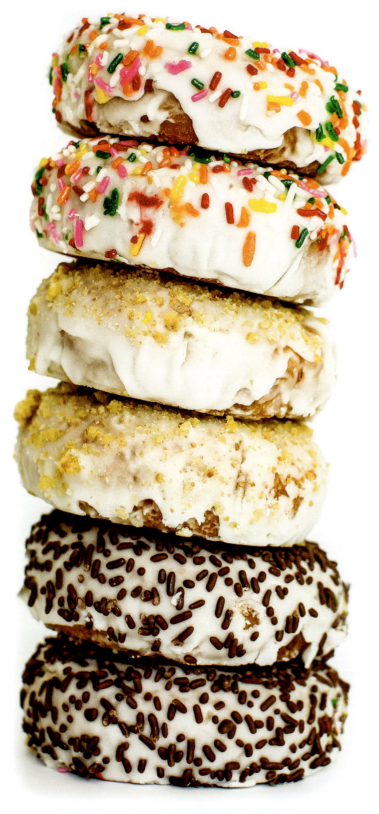

Fear Of Missing Out

Although you might have excitement when beginning a diet and the changes it might bring about, there is also immediate FOMO involved: "fear of missing out." The struggle is real. In ONE-TWO PUNCH nothing is removed or cut out. You're making a choice about WHICH protein and WHICH carbohydrate. That fist of protein can be a lovely piece of grilled salmon and the fist of carb can be brown-rice pilaf. Or, the protein fist can be two sausage links and the carb fist a cupcake.

I like to say there's no wagon to fall off of when practicing ONE-TWO PUNCH. There are just different choices. When eating within the suggestions of OTP, there's no guilt and no shame. You solved your physical hunger and ate what sounded good. So now let's move on.

When you eat something appealing, you are sensually satisfied as well. This means it was pleasurable in addition to fulfilling a physical need.

I can solve ANYONE's physical hunger with a piece of boiled meat and a stale piece of bread. But that person will still be sensually hungry because they didn't have something enjoyable and satisfying to their soul and brain.[13-14]

For this to work, in order for ONE-TWO PUNCH to be sustainable, you HAVE to give yourself permission to have the foods you love. I differ from some colleagues when I say you should NEVER, EVER eat anything you don't like. EVER.

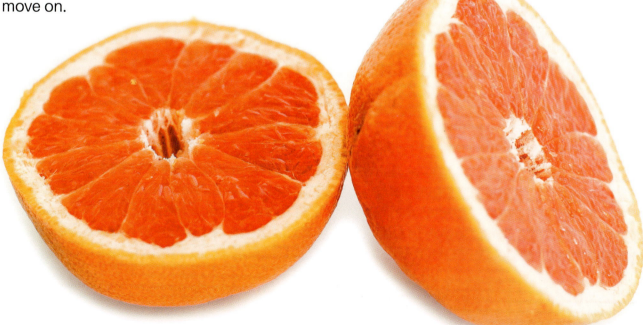

If you really don't like vegetables, we can get around that. Don't eat something you don't like. Just don't. Period. It won't be sustainable. It breeds feelings of deprivation. Sensual satisfaction is as important as solving physical hunger. We all have a need to be sensually satisfied with food.[14]

ONE-TWO PUNCH gives you permission not to have to choke down something you simply don't enjoy. Permission is a very necessary step in this whole process. Sure, you can have the salmon and brown-rice pilaf with a pile of salad. You don't need me or this book to tell you that it's healthy. But if that's not what you like or crave, how long do you think that practice is going to last? And you're likely miserable for the entire time that it does manage to last.

You cannot skip the permission step. You can't skip over all the yummy foods you love and jump right to eating whole, natural, "clean" foods. What you've skipped over, or tried to, is deprivation. It comes back to bite you in the butt. Because you're feeling deprived (mad, sad, lots of FOMO), you're likely to overeat the "healthy" foods instead of focusing on the first foundational principle of ONE-TWO PUNCH: BURN.

It doesn't work to just eat as much as you want of only healthy foods. Ask anyone who's tried it. Eventually, you realize that you have to eat within the structure of what your body can handle — the incinerator. Or, you realize that it can't be sustained because you can't stay away from the brownies for the rest of your life. And then because of that, you throw in the towel and eat the rest of the pan of brownies. Oh, little by little, of course... just one more sliver. You know the drill.

And, if you've gone through enough deprivation, the body tries to make up for lost time. Ever wonder how long your "off-the-wagon" time will last? Possibly as long as the deprivation has lasted. Oooooh, that's a sobering thought, isn't it? The permission section is an excellent place to quote a famous food author: "Absolutism in the quest for food is a huge mistake," said Michael Pollan in his approach to being a happy and healthy eater.[79] With ONE-TWO PUNCH,

> With ONE-TWO PUNCH, you're not depriving yourself; you're making choices.

you're not depriving yourself; you're making choices.

Does balancing protein and carbohydrate mean that you will always have to have one bite of chicken breast and then one bite of cheesecake every time you want it? No. Your stomach and your digestive system don't work that quickly, thank goodness!!! It does mean making decisions. If you know there's cheesecake or (insert your favorite treat) available, you make a decision to have that as your carbohydrate. Maybe you have grilled chicken over a salad or steamed vegetables with a steak and then your treat as your carb. Enjoy it, and call it a day! Rather, just call it a yummy meal and wait until the next time your incinerator door is open – the next time you get hungry.

Permission indeed makes a big difference. Don't skip over it and try to forget that you EVER wanted a cupcake, or candy bar, or key lime pie or donut. You can't justify eating more than the size of your fist just because you're eating healthy foods. You still have to honor the first foundational principle, which is physical hunger and need. Sure you might really, really WANT a particular food, but that's very different than NEED as we discussed in the last section.

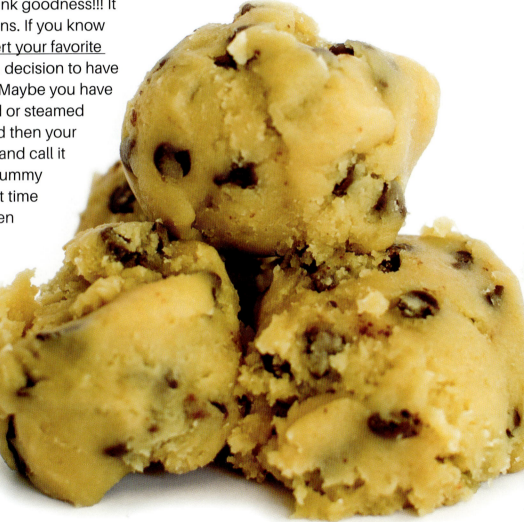

This could be you!

I was diagnosed with Polycystic Ovarian Syndrome (PCOS) in my early twenties. Although I did not experience many of the extreme weight loss/gain issues that other PCOS people experience, my appetite changed. I constantly felt hungry and never fully satisfied. I have always been very active, but when I started training for my first half marathon, I got so frustrated with myself because I never seemed to have enough energy to make it through.

When I wasn't making progress with fitness, I felt frustrated because I didn't think I looked fit. This made me think that I needed to eat less food, or eat smaller portions in order to get the results I wanted, which of course left me weak, hungry and unsatisfied. This tug-of-war between fitness and food was a constant battle of pushing myself to look and feel fit while trying to satisfy my body's need for nutrition.

When I tried to get control of this battle, I started following a diet and fitness plan (21 Day Fix) that focused on portion control and color-coded food containers. At first, this felt great because it was something tangible that was supposed to help me understand different types of foods and the appropriate portion and times to have them. But I found myself even more frustrated because, being gluten and dairy intolerant, I was so limited by my options. I remember finishing a tough workout looking in the refrigerator in tears because I was so weak and hungry but couldn't find anything to eat that would meet the requirements of my plan.

My first breakthrough with ONE-TWO PUNCH happened during my first meeting with Claudia when she helped me to understand that when I experience hunger it is my body telling me it needs to be filled up. When I fill it with an unbalanced meal like an apple, it is not really being filled up and will naturally be empty again. Understanding hunger and how to balance meals was the first key to success for me. It was so freeing to recognize when I was really hungry, I could fill my body with what seemed appetizing to me. As long as I had a fist of protein and a fist of carbohydrate I knew I was balanced.

My second breakthrough happened over time as I continued to practice OTP. Understanding balanced nutrition has helped me to understand balance in other areas of my life as well. There is something psychological that happens when I eat a balanced meal, I don't feel so much pressure to work out extra hard at the gym to compensate for a large meal from the day before. I don't feel this constant, unsettled, unsatisfied feeling that lead me to seek out satisfaction from other things. And I handle stress in a much healthier way because I understand how it affects my body. ONE-TWO PUNCH has changed everything for me!

-Noelle

Don't eat anything you don't like. Just don't.

"THE DEVIL IS IN THE DETAILS"

The idiom "the devil is in the details" means that mistakes are usually made in the small details of a project. Usually it is a caution to pay attention to details to avoid failure. I use the phrase in the opposite way: If you get too bogged down in the details of ONE-TWO PUNCH, you will drive yourself crazy. It will then become just like any other diet that ends up not being sustainable. The "devil" is found in making this process too detailed and in over-analyzing your food choices.

One of the reasons diets aren't sustainable is that the process is working against you. While exciting at first, all the planning, tracking, measuring, weighing, reading labels and calculating is causing additional stress. Remember when you increase your stress you increase cortisol levels in your body and increased cortisol levels increase your potential to store fat.[35] We need to cut out the stress! ONE-TWO PUNCH is designed to reduce the stress of eating and help you eat in a balanced way.

Balance also means balance in the foods you choose to eat. Yes, the fist of carb can be anything, but do we want it to be a brownie every single time, every single day? No. Balance means, for the most part, you are choosing foods in the whole, unprocessed, unrefined form; foods with the fewest ingredients on the nutrition label. But balance also means choosing a Twinkie (think heavily processed) occasionally when it sounds good to you. If you need to think of that balance in more tangible terms, think of an 80/20% rule:

- 80% of the time you are choosing foods with more fiber, more water content, more protein, stronger flavors and less processing. Generally speaking, these foods tend to be more satisfying, have more nutrients and keep you full longer.

- 20% of the time you are choosing foods with taste and enjoyment as a priority, not the actual content of the food. These foods, while perhaps nutritionally lacking, can be highly satisfying and make you crave less.

Yes, to be successful at maintaining a healthy weight, the number of calories consumed and the quality of those calories matter. What I'm advocating is that if you eat only when you are hungry, the calories you consume will fall in line to match what your body needs. Even if you allow treats, you are still eating when your body will burn them. I call high-sugar foods, like candy, intense carbohydrates. By giving yourself permission to have treats in a balanced way, you'll stop the yo-yo action of going on and off various diets.

You want a balance between protein and carbohydrate, but also a balance between ridiculously healthy and just outright deliciousness, caution thrown to the wind regarding ingredients.[32,80] The next section will help you practice your balancing act.

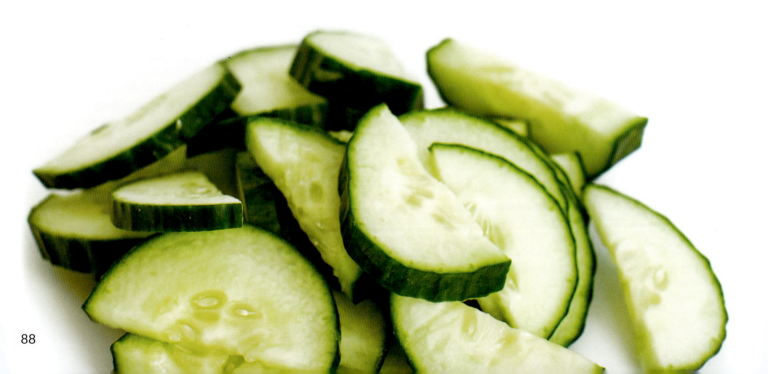

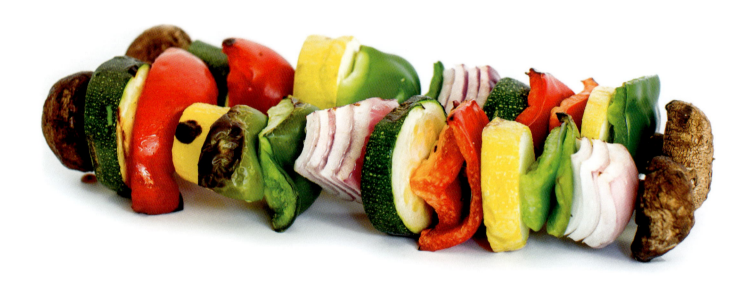

BECOME

This principle is putting into practice the first two components, BURN and BALANCE. It is practicing. You are building a skill that over time becomes easier and easier. To maintain a skill, you must continue to practice. Practice is an ongoing process that really never ends; there's no "arrival." It reflects a change in lifestyle.

Not having an endpoint can make it hard to understand this process; there's no destination except that you learn how to aptly eat for hunger and fullness and balance your intake in order to maintain a healthy body and healthy weight.

BECOME is the practice of sensing hunger, balancing protein and carbohydrate and choosing the options that are most helpful to you and the circumstance. It is an active process, not necessarily an end goal you achieve. You are increasingly working to BECOME the YOU you've always wanted to be.

To become means to change and develop into a person who eats in a healthy and balanced way, both physically and mentally. Live your life, create your surroundings, do your thing, engage in your work, participate in whatever it is that you are doing at the present moment — all the things that make up your days. Just BE and let the hunger signal come to you. Let it interrupt whatever it is you are doing.

For some people, the HARDEST work of this process is finding the life they love, the activities they enjoy. In doing this work, they realize that they were eating when they weren't hungry because they actually weren't engaged in things they enjoyed. It is sometimes easy to want to take a break from something you don't like. It's easy to use the excuse of eating to take that break. When you are engaged in something you enjoy, you're more likely to be interrupted by your hunger.

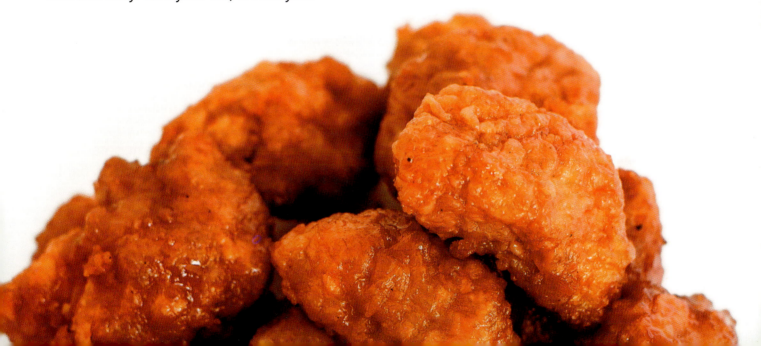

Of course you can't only do things you love all the time. There are things that have to be done in life — paying taxes comes to mind. But if most of your time and most of your days are filled with things you don't enjoy, and you're eating because of it, it will be harder to sit through those things without eating as a way of taking a break.

Practice is allowing your body to function naturally. It is learning the trust fall with your body signals and your ability to experience them and respond to them. It is you being you and letting your body do it's own thing. I know this might be different from anything you've ever heard.

You've mostly heard that to be an appropriate weight and be healthy you have to take charge and follow a plan. When you operate in that space, you are acknowledging that food has all the power and that you need to control it. It is really YOU that has all the power; you just need to recognize it and put food back in its place.

To practice or BECOME is also taking ONE-TWO PUNCH to a point where it works for you. That is the point that feels most comfortable for the longest period of time. Do you feel better eating "cleanly" with lots of vegetables, fruits and grains in their natural form with minimal processing? Do you notice a difference eating organic meats? For ethical or personal reasons do you choose to be vegan or vegetarian? You can take ONE-TWO PUNCH in any direction, while keeping in mind that sometimes you have a "less healthy" treat because the situation warrants it. A warranted situation might simply be because you want it.

You don't need me to tell you what foods are healthier than others. I've searched and searched to find the original author of this quote. If you're reading this book and you think it's you, contact me! I absolutely love it and it aptly applies here: "Some days you eat salads and go to the gym; some days you eat cupcakes and refuse to put on pants. It's called balance." I do think this process allows us to have it all.

> Practice is allowing your body to function naturally.

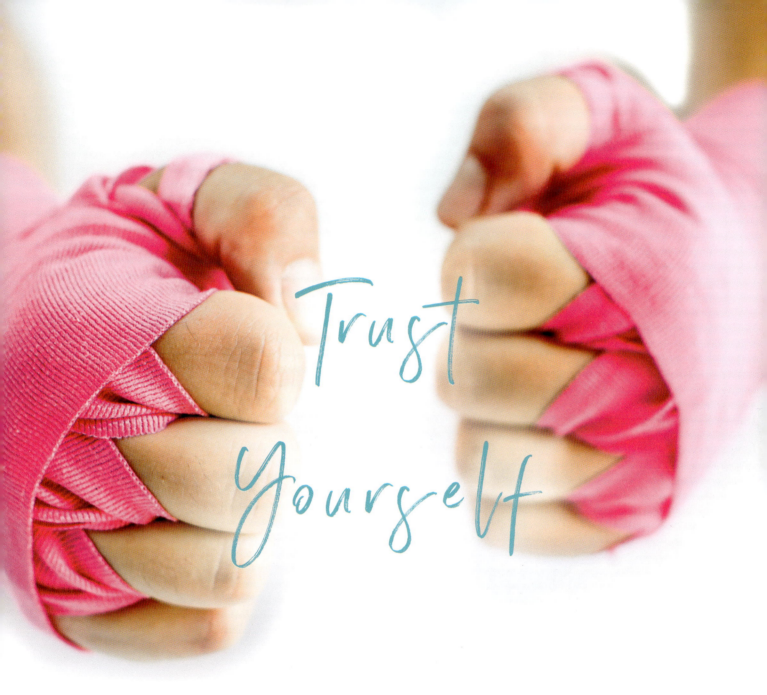

This could be you! →

After having kids my body changed; my mental health changed. I found myself exhausted in a way I didn't know and fulfilled in a way I didn't know. In an attempt to go back to what I was and what I thought my body should be I tried every way to eat – elimination diets, measuring food, ordering expensive shakes. I paid a lot of money per month for a protein shake that was going to help me lose weight and use all these containers and stuff. And, ya, I totally lost weight and I definitely felt better.

The problem came when it wasn't sustainable. I don't have time to measure out how much fruit I'm eating if I'm packing two lunches, getting kids to daycare and going to work. It wasn't possible.

ONE-TWO PUNCH helped me learn to trust myself again. It helped me trust when I'm actually hungry or recognize that I'm sad or that I'm overwhelmed as a mom or I'm happy, but that doesn't mean I need to eat all the cake at my kids' birthday party to deal with it. In reality I need to know whether or not I am hungry; whether or not I am doing okay. If I am hungry, now I know what to eat. I can choose.

My refrigerator and pantry are stocked with healthy foods that make me feel good. But they are also stocked with Peanut M&M's and I don't feel bad about it anymore. I've adjusted my eating times to know what sustains me instead of eating according to what I thought was the perfect time. I learned there was no perfect time to eat – I needed to eat when I was hungry. ONE-TWO PUNCH also helped me deal with guilt. I need to eat according to what's good for me instead of how Suzie Q is eating. We all have different bodies and different needs and OTP helped me come to terms with that.

—Claire

PRACTICE HUNGER

Wouldn't it be great if your stomach was equipped with a visual gauge, similar to the gas gauge in your car? That way your body would tell you exactly how many calories you need in order to gain, lose or maintain your weight. That's exactly what most diet programs aim to do. They act as an external gas gauge and tell you when to fill the tank, what to fill it with and how soon to come back to the tank again.

Diet plans provide a template of how, what and when to eat, but they are regimented. It's possible to develop an internal, virtual type of gas gauge for you to sense hunger that is more flexible.

The ability to feel hunger and fullness is a sensation that you were born with.[81] So in a sense, you were born with a gauge. As you mature, this ability sometimes goes awry—you learn to ignore it, confuse it with thirst or emotion and may eventually forget it altogether. It becomes too hard to see or sense the gauge so you rely on external templates, like diets, to perform the function of the gauge.

There is a tool that can help you tune into your hunger and fullness gauge so you

HUNGER/FULLNESS SCALE									
1	2	3	4	5	6	7	8	9	10
Starving, weak, dizzy	Very hungry, low energy, stomach growling a lot	Pretty hungry, stomach is growling	Starting to feel a little hungry	Satisfied, neither hungry nor full	A little full, pleasantly full	A little uncomfortable	Feeling stuffed	Very uncomfortable stomach hurts	So full I feel sick

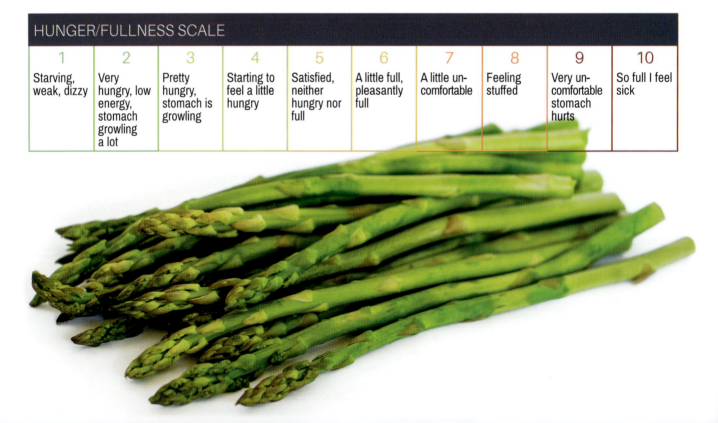

don't overfill your belly or wait too long to eat between meals. You can actually train yourself to tune into your ability to feel hunger and fullness by visualizing a Hunger Scale.[12,82-83]

You can obtain a virtual fuel gauge through practice and development of a new skill. The tank I want you to envision is your incinerator, your stomach. Imagine a meter ranging from 0-10, with 0 being empty and 10 being so full it's actually bulging. While everyone has their own definitions, physical experiences and symptoms of what hunger and fullness feel like, there are some generalities.

There are varying degrees of hunger. You might be really hungry or only a little hungry. If you are a little hungry and want to eat, this would be a time to have half of a fist-sized portion of protein and a corresponding half fist of carbohydrate.

A situation in which you might find this helpful is when you are dining with others. Suppose you're meeting friends for dinner in a couple of hours, but you're hungry now. Not hungry enough to eat a full fist of protein and a full fist of carbohydrates, but hungry enough not to want to wait. And you don't want to feel like eating your dinner mates as you look over a menu! This would be a time to have a smaller portion of protein and carbohydrate; think of a half fist of each.

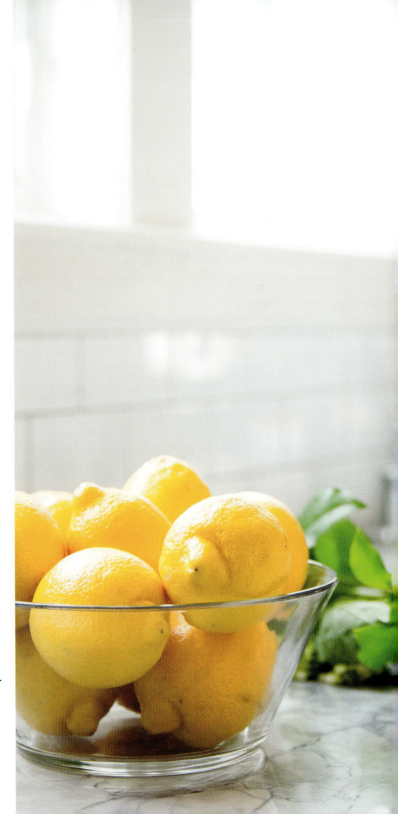

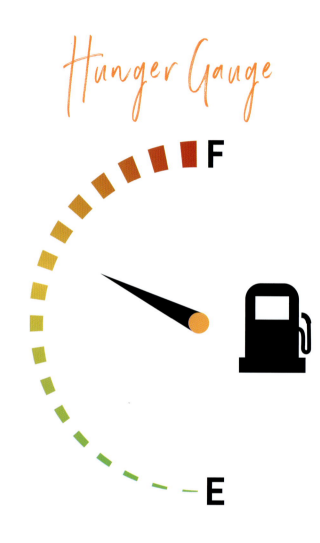

Hunger Gauge

0 - EMPTY
ANYTHING! You'll eat anything and actually you want EVERYTHING! You want it all and then some. And you feel like adding extra (probably sweet stuff) for good measure. You feel crazed probably because you have low blood sugar and you feel dizzy, lightheaded and pissed at the world in general.

1 - NEARLY EMPTY
Your energy level is low and productivity is down. You probably feel shaky, have poor concentration and your mood is declining.

2 - REALLY HUNGRY
Your stomach feels empty and hollow and food is dominating your thoughts. You need to find some food fast and your energy levels are dropping. Junk food is starting to sound very appealing.

3 - HUNGRY
You can tell, within your body, it's time to eat. If you wait any longer you're going to start feeling physical symptoms that aren't pleasant; symptoms that biologically you try to avoid.

4 - SLIGHTLY HUNGRY
You're starting to think about your next meal. You could eat, but could also wait a bit. If you ate now, you'd probably only want a little.

5 - NEUTRAL
You are neither hungry nor full. You're just doing your thing (whatever that is) and not thinking about food.

6 - SLIGHTLY SATISFIED
The hunger sensation is gone. There is food in your belly, but you could definitely eat more. If you stopped now, you would probably be hungry again soon.

7 - SATISFIED
Hunger sensation is long gone. You could eat more because it's so comforting or because it tastes amazing or because it's one of your favorites. You feel content and satisfied and don't need to eat more.

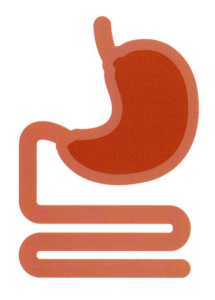

8 - FULL
You were perfectly content and then pushed the envelope just a little. Those last three to four bites put you over the edge. If you're wearing something tight around your belly, you want to loosen it a bit.

9 - NEARLY UNCOMFORTABLE
You overate and your stomach feels overfull. You're finding it a little hard to breathe; you have to really concentrate and it's a little painful and maybe a little nauseating. You do not want to talk about food.

10 - STUFFED
Oh wow. You went waaaay too far. You feel like the kid in the movie "A Christmas Story" wearing a constricting snow suit that allows little movement. You definitely need some comfy clothes, but you're finding it hard to move, let alone breathe. Lying down is worse; you need to be propped up a bit.

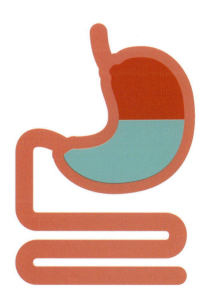

How to Respond to Physical Hunger

1

If you've already determined you are hungry, **rank your hunger on the scale before you start to eat**. Practice the paced eating tips in this section to really evaluate how you are moving through the different numbers on the hunger scale.

2

Halfway through your meal, rank your hunger again using the scale. Keep in mind that the difference between each number on the scale may only be a few bites.

3

At the end of your planned meal rank your hunger again for practice and evaluation. What did you like about it? What do you wish was different? What would you do next time? Do you feel you went too far? If so, why? Don't judge, just gather data for the future. Did you enjoy it so much that you didn't want to stop? Or did you start out way too hungry, so you couldn't pay attention? When that happens all bets are off. Reason and health go out the window and it's survival mode for your physical body.

HOW TO RESPOND TO PHYSICAL HUNGER

If you are in the habit of planning out times to eat and eating on a schedule, you are in a sense using some type of visible gas gauge and may not be ready to trust yourself internally. If eating has been chaotic and haphazard, hunger and fullness hormones are going to be unreliable.

If you've been severely restricting your calories for a long time or you've been yo-yo dieting and going through periods of binge eating, it will be difficult to determine true hunger and fullness because those signals are out of whack. Those innate senses have been turned off and ignored for too long and they need to be brought back to life.[12] For these reasons, waiting until you feel the internal hunger signal can be unsettling and unstable.

Until you're ready to wait for hunger to happen, having structured times set during the day to check in with yourself can feel more supportive. Checking in every 2-3 hours to see how you feel, and choosing to eat even if you're not sure you're hungry, might feel safer. With practice, and by balancing your carbohydrates and protein at every meal and snack, a continuous rhythm will develop that normalizes your hormones and allows you to wait until your incinerator door truly opens.

You can hit the reset button through eating balanced meals of protein, carbohydrate and fat. See section on BALANCE. You can do this by using fist-sized portions and following a pattern of eating every 3-5 hours. It's important that you try to understand how you're feeling before, during and after those planned meals as you practice recognizing the signals. Practicing in this way will help your body get back in tune with a rhythmic pattern of eating that allows normal peaks and valleys in satiety.

The next page shows the difference between eating according to times versus eating according to your physical hunger. Whether you eat at specified times or wait for your physical hunger signal, the food could be the same. However, as we have discussed, it is more effective to eat when physically hungry, when your body incinerator is going to BURN it.

An omnivore and vegan plan demonstrate how you might balance your fist-sized portion of protein and carbohydrate every time you eat, regardless of the foods you choose.

When to Eat

A *traditional plan* frequently gives times for meals and snacks. For instance, eating breakfast at 7:00am and lunch at noon.

A plan based on your *physical hunger* uses your body signals to determine when to eat a meal or snack.

The food you are eating on either plan is the same. The difference is eating by the clock instead of eating according to physical hunger.

It is more effective to eat when physically hungry because your body will use the food more readily.

TRADITIONAL PLAN	PHYSICAL HUNGER PLAN
BREAKFAST	1ST HUNGER
SNACK	2ND HUNGER
LUNCH	3RD HUNGER
SNACK	4TH HUNGER
DINNER	5TH HUNGER
SNACK	6TH HUNGER

Omnivore Meal Plan

MONDAY	TUESDAY	WEDNESDAY	THURSDAY	FRIDAY	SATURDAY
1 egg 1 pc ham tortilla	2 eggs 2 waffles	1 cup oatmeal handful nuts	veggie omelette toast	1 egg 1 pc ham English muffin	French toast
cheese stick apple	Greek yogurt plum	hard-boiled egg crackers	jerky apple	handful nuts orange	cheese stick nectarine
turkey sandwich veggies	grilled steak salad 2 small rolls	chicken sandwich cucumber slices	turkey sandwich	ham wrap	tofu noodle bowl
handful almonds banana	cottage cheese strawberries	Greek yogurt raspberries	cheese slices plum	cottage cheese crackers	flavored Greek yogurt
steak sweet potato salad	BBQ chicken rice broccoli	turkey burger salad	marinara pasta w/ turkey burger	tofu teriyaki stir fry rice	grilled salmon potatoes asparagus
Greek yogurt orange	edamame rice crackers	cottage cheese peach	Greek yogurt 2 cups popcorn	smoothie	cottage cheese mixed berries

When to Eat

A *traditional plan* frequently gives times for meals and snacks. For instance, eating breakfast at 7:00am and lunch at noon.

A plan based on your *physical hunger* uses your body signals to determine when to eat a meal or snack.

The food you are eating on either plan is the same. The difference is eating by the clock instead of eating according to physical hunger.

It is more effective to eat when physically hungry because your body will use the food more readily.

TRADITIONAL PLAN	PHYSICAL HUNGER PLAN
BREAKFAST	1ST HUNGER
SNACK	2ND HUNGER
LUNCH	3RD HUNGER
SNACK	4TH HUNGER
DINNER	5TH HUNGER
SNACK	6TH HUNGER

Vegan Meal Plan

MONDAY	TUESDAY	WEDNESDAY	THURSDAY	FRIDAY	SATURDAY
oatmeal with protein powder	vegan protein bar	tofu scramble	vegan protein bar	tofu scramble	oatmeal protein pancakes
almonds fruit	soy yogurt strawberries	vegan cheese crackers	almond butter fruit	cashews orange	almonds fruit
hummus vegetables	lentil soup	vegan wrap	lentil soup	veggie burger bun	vegan cheese crackers
cashew butter apple	vegan cheese fruit	coconut yogurt raspberries	trail mix	hummus vegetables	protein powder shake
salad rice & beans tofu	tofu rice broccoli	tempeh steak quinoa	seitan sandwich	vegan macaroni and cheese	tofu new potatoes asparagus
almond yogurt orange	vegan dessert	vegan proetin powder shake	vegan dessert	cashew yogurt frozen berries	vegan dessert

PRACTICE EMOTIONS

As we discussed in the BURN section, sometimes the emotions that hit you in your core can make it very, very difficult to detect what's really going on. Identifying feelings other than hunger is going to take practice. Lots and lots of practice. This section is going to help you with that.

Over time with that practice you will be able to distinguish emotional hunger from physical hunger. It can be tricky because emotional hunger can totally feel physical. Totally. You're normal. I'm still going to use the words emotional and physical to distinguish the two.[8,13-14,84] Let's start with the graph below.

	Emotional Hunger	*Physical Hunger*
WHERE	Chest Upper diaphragm (both sides)	Stomach Body weakness
TIMING	Feels urgent Evening, when tired Feels strong, but you're full	Fairly predictable About 3-5 hours since last balanced meal
FOOD TYPE	Highly specific food craving	Open to many different options
COMPANY	Frequently alone	In view of others

Now let's practice by following this exercise as you start thinking about getting food:

Each time you reach for something to eat, go to the fridge, the pantry, the cupboard, leave your desk, walk to the kitchen, go to the employee break room, reach in your desk drawer, ask yourself this question: "What am I feeling right now?"

You need to figure out what's making you seek food. Sure, it might be hunger, but you might also recognize that you are reaching for food in the absence of physical hunger. If so, why? Keep in mind that if you are willing to explore and sit with the results, you might notice that you are discovering emotions that you didn't know were there.

You might also notice that some of the emotions that you knew were there are feeling more intense now that you are not covering them up with food. This is normal. And it can also be scary.

Lots of people who enter this process are not even aware that they are eating when an uncomfortable feeling comes up. They don't know why they're eating. That's called mindless eating. Asking yourself WHY you are eating is designed to increase your awareness. There are SO many feelings to feel and explore. It can be overwhelming.

As we've discussed, there are other body sensations that, while real, may not be true stomach hunger. Examples of "false alarms" include the following:

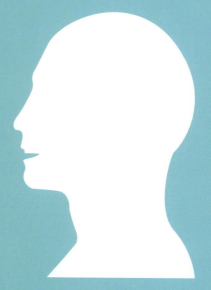

Teeth Hunger
Irritation and frustration can increase an urge to chew the stress away to relieve anxiety.

Mouth Hunger
A desire for the taste of food (aka, a little party in your mouth) can bring on a craving, and seeing or smelling a tasty treat can make your mouth start to water.

Brain Hunger
Most people are well conditioned and trained to think in terms of "lunch time" or "dinner time." You may look at the clock and think it's time regardless of how your stomach feels.

Identifying Physical Hunger

Here are some questions that may help you practice identifying and recognizing your physical hunger:

- What are your physical signs of hunger?

- When was the last time you ate?

- Where are you on the hunger scale?

- What are you wanting/feeling if it is not hunger?

- What would happen if you sat with this feeling?

- How long can you tolerate this feeling?

- Do you understand this feeling?

Exploring Emotions/Feelings

Here are some questions that may help you practice exploring the emotions/feelings that you might be mistaking as physical hunger:

- Where is the desire to eat coming from?

- What were you feeling before you were prompted to eat?

- What is going on with you right now?

- What is the most important thing going on in your life currently?

- What, other than food, would satisfy your emotional need?

- What scares you the most about this feeling?

- What do you really want?

Sometimes you feel an ache or emptiness in your heart or soul due to a recent loss or ongoing, unmet emotional or spiritual need. It's easy to mistake this for physical need and try to fill the void with food. Or you use food to "stuff" your feelings deeper so that you don't feel them quite as painfully. There is definitely a physical discomfort in the gut, but it is a different sensation from stomach hunger.

If you want to explore why you want to eat when you're not physically hungry, it's a good idea to record/journal/text how you feel before, during and after eating. If you find that you're resistant to journaling before you eat, as many people are, begin by journaling after every eating experience. Ask yourself why you just ate (fill in the blank) .

You can take this practice one step further by tracking things like energy, mood,

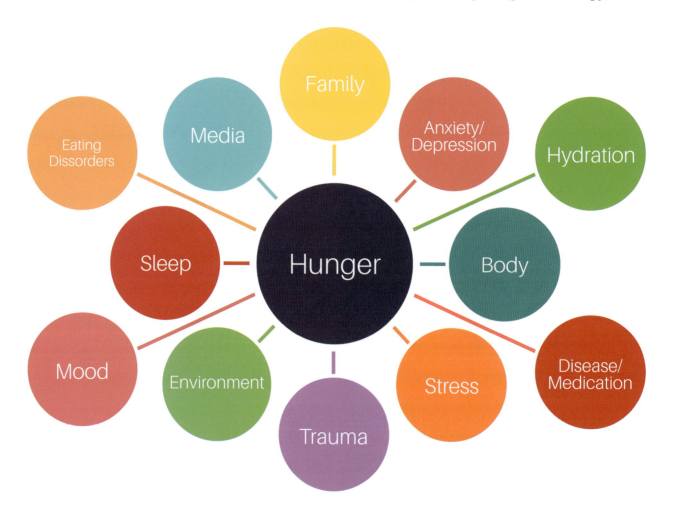

mental clarity and digestive happiness. Record how the food feels in your stomach and body.

In your exploration you might discover times when you are not physically hungry, but you can't identify or pinpoint the feeling. You might also find that you know you are not physically hungry, but also not ready to dive in and process the emotion that you discovered. Both situations are okay and with practice you will be able to identify the emotion and start to explore it further.

One of the most challenging times you might face in deciphering your physical hunger is when you're not sure. Could be yes, could be no. Can I get a maybe? One tip: if you are not sure, chances are high that you are not actually physically hungry.

In wading through the yes, no or maybe, I suggest making a list of your top three "go-tos" to engage you while you wait to be sure of hunger. They have to be quick, accessible and easy. The idea is to first hydrate yourself, so you cover the possibility of only being thirsty, then busy yourself with something fun and stimulating for a few minutes.

If your stomach interrupts the activity you choose, there's a good chance you are definitely physically hungry. Remember it has to be something you like to do. It's easy to want a break when doing un-fun chores. I imagine I would want a break if I were vacuuming, for instance!

I'm encouraging you to take a fun break instead of turning to food, even when all the work isn't done. Here's my list of go-tos:

1. Drink 16oz or more of water. Yes, I pee a TON and have no sympathy for you!

2. Search something fun, non-work related on the internet. Pop culture fascinates me as it distracts me from reality and lets me fantasize about being discovered by a celebrity.

3. Search fun, new accounts to follow on Instagram.

There are so many things you can allow yourself, or reward yourself with, without turning to food. I've given you my list. What would you do for 5-10 minutes if you had nothing to do? If all your responsibilities were taken care of and your work was done?

Here's another way I reward myself. I love magazines — I love the pictures, the articles, the quotes, the colors, the different fonts, the clothes (especially those), the ads, the whole spread. I love them. I try to set boundaries for myself around this activity. Before I indulge, I try to be reasonably caught up on work and things around the house. There are always things I can do. Is reading the magazines a waste of time? Perhaps. But it brings me a bit of frivolous joy.

Maybe frivolous joy to you includes some of the things I've mentioned above or it's a bubble bath, pedicure, zoning out with Netflix, coloring, knitting or a simple game on your phone. Okay, some of these take more than 10 minutes. My point is these little pleasures are not frivolous. Think of them as how you recover from the demands of your life, how you refuel yourself emotionally and

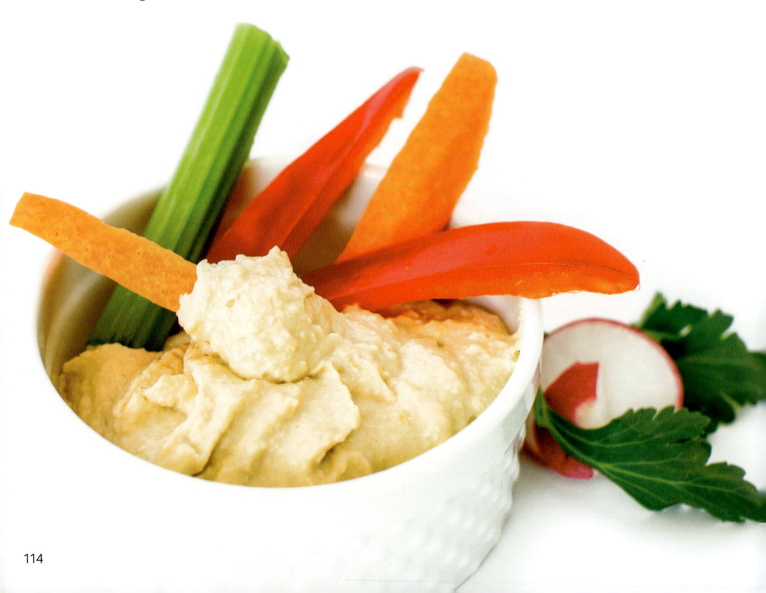

give yourself a little present for doing the best you can.

Many people often use food as the frivolous joy; a little food present as a reward. However, some of the side effects of eating more than you need are not rewarding! If you are in the habit of eating when you are not hungry, as a way of managing your life, to have a little "party in your mouth" as stimulation, wouldn't it be better to allow yourself 5-10 minutes of non-food frivolous joy? Even if everything else isn't done? You feel me?

PRACTICE WITH FULLNESS

There's lots of material out there on mindful eating. I call it "being with your food" and only your food. If you've never eaten without any other distractions, all by yourself, it can be an eerie experience.

In non-distracted eating, the idea is to limit the distractions and variables that keep you from totally focusing on your eating experience. You want to set yourself up for success in deciphering what's happening with your food and in your body. To do that you need to prepare. I suggest very concrete ways of cutting out the distractions while eating so you have the best possible chance to detect fullness when it happens.

Non-Distracted Eating

- Always sit down

- Put food containers away

- Use plates, bowls and utensils

- No computer

- No phone

- No TV

- No book, magazine or newspaper

- Don't eat while driving

- Stop eating if conversation around you becomes too distracting and/or too engaging

Paced Eating

1. Get your first bite ready (food on fork or sandwich in hand for instance)

2. Take a bite

3. Set utensil or food down; let go of it and sit back

4. Finish eating and swallowing completely the first bite before getting the next bite ready

5. Breathe while chewing

6. Sit back from the table and sit up straight while chewing

I also suggest very defined ways of pacing yourself as you eat. I call it paced eating — inserting pause points for you to check in with yourself while eating to keep the momentum of the meal from going too fast.

By inserting pause points while eating you will be more aware and more mindful of the sensations in your stomach and when you feel satisfied. Pause points will also prolong the eating experience and allow your stomach to signal to your brain that you've eaten.

This will promote feeling full before mistakenly overeating and overstuffing the incinerator.[85] Eating with pause points uses the 20-30 minutes it takes to register the eating experience in your mind.[21,86]

Okay, so you've tried all that. You even went to your three trusted go-tos, but you still want to keep eating and you don't know why. However, you know it's not physical hunger. It can be helpful to understand the reasons why the desire persists.

Sometimes it's the set-up that leads us to keep wanting more. It's going to take practice to understand the reasons.

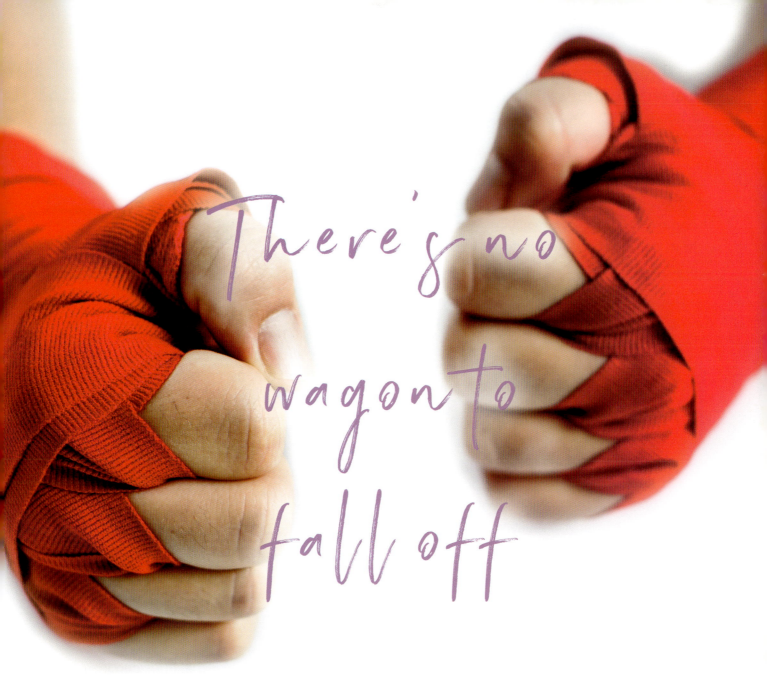

Here are some examples of situations that set you up for wanting to eat more, even when you know you are physically full:

You chose something you really didn't want.

As I mentioned, satisfaction doesn't just come from being physically full but also from being sensually satisfied, meaning you enjoyed what you ate.

- You can prevent this by exploring what you really want before you eat. This is where choosing ANY fist of protein and ANY fist of carb, regardless of how healthy it seems, can be helpful.

- If you realize part way through eating that you don't really like what you're eating or you're not enjoying it, stop. Switch to something else or decide to wait until the next time you're hungry to get what you really want.

- If you realize you don't like what you're eating, but there are no other options, decide that you will get something you love the next time it's possible.

You were distracted while eating.

If you weren't paying attention to your food and instead were focused on the gripping movie you were watching, your brain didn't get to enjoy the food — it was watching the movie!! You might be physically full, but the eating experience didn't really register. Practicing non-distracted and paced eating tips help avoid this.

You were eating something extraordinary.

In other words, you were eating something that you don't normally eat or have access to. Fear that you won't get that particular food again can bring about feelings of future deprivation that can promote overeating to "store up" the experience.

While you might not be able to have that exact food again, such as when you're visiting a country that you likely won't visit again, think about how you might recreate the experience at another time when you are hungry. You might think about learning to make the food or checking your local neighborhood for similar foods.

You were triggered by environmental cues.

The following external cues can lead to overeating: too much food on your plate, not wanting to waste food, eating to get your money's worth (think all-you-can-eat buffets),

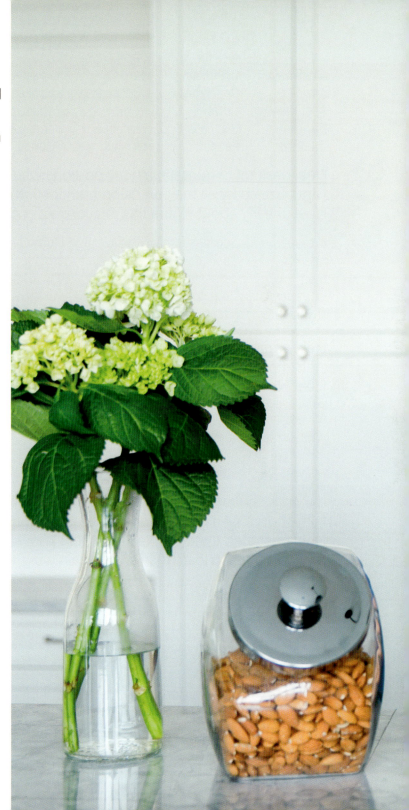

trying to fit in and keep up with your fellow eaters and so many more!! ONE-TWO PUNCH can help you visualize what and how much you are eating so the outside distractions can be shut down.

You were responding to an emotion.

When a craving or drive to eat doesn't come from physical hunger, eating won't satisfy it. You will want to keep eating, thinking that at some point it will be enough. But, you weren't hungry in the first place.

Eating has served as a distraction, but you are still left with the boredom, stress, loneliness, frustration, sadness that was present when you began. To prevent this it's important to resist eating when you know you're not physically hungry and search for something else to respond to the emotion.

Check out the feeling lists in this section to help in your exploration of emotions. They are categorized into four generally titled sections, but I think you'll see that not every emotion fits neatly within a category.

For instance, is "shocked" an exact feeling of anger? Is "ambivalent" an exact feeling of afraid? The categories are meant to guide you as you search and explore your emotions. Don't get caught up in where a particular emotion fits.

AFRAID

Ambivalent	Confused	Frantic	Insecure	Puzzled	Shy	Uneasy
Anxious	Concerned	Frightened	Panicked	Rattled	Suspicious	Worried
Apprehensive	Cowardly	Frozen	Paranoid	Restless	Stunned	
Bewildered	Disoriented	Hesitant	Perplexed	Reluctant	Threatened	
Cautious	Fearful	Horrified	Petrified	Scared	Timid	

I feel hesitant to guesstimate my portions without measuring my food.
I am puzzled by all the confusing nutrition information out there.
I feel uneasy about where this relationship is going.

GLAD

Amazed	Confident	Ecstatic	Hopeful	Mellow	Playful	Satisfied
Amused	Content	Exhilarated	Important	Mischievous	Protective	Sympathetic
Calm	Determined	Free	Joyous	Nurturing	Proud	
Cherished	Delighted	Fulfilled	Loving	Optimistic	Relieved	
Comfortable	Eager	Happy	Loose	Peaceful	Respected	

I feel comfortable with the choices I made for lunch.
I felt important when a colleague asked for my opinion.
I feel playful when I'm joking around with friends.

MAD

Abused	Appalled	Disapproving	Frustrated	Impatient	Negative	Stubborn
Aggressive	Blamed	Disgusted	Furious	Indifferent	Ornery	Victimized
Alienated	Bitter	Enraged	Guilty	Irritated	Resentful	
Angry	Bored	Envious	Hostile	Lethargic	Shocked	
Apathetic	Controlled	Exasperated	Horrified	Manipulated	Smothered	

I am angry that a friend canceled on me at the last minute.
I feel frustrated that I keep eating after I know I'm full.
I was shocked to learn that I didn't gain weight after not measuring my food.

SAD

Abandoned	Disappointed	Empty	Humiliated	Jinxed	Overlooked	Worthless
Agonized	Discouraged	Foolish	Hurt	Lonely	Regretful	Vulnerable
Apologetic	Disregarded	Forgotten	Hysterical	Lost	Rejected	
Burdened	Distant	Grief	Impotent	Miserable	Upset	
Desperate	Embarrassed	Hopeless	Isolated	Neglected	Withdrawn	

I sometimes feel burdened by my responsibilities as a parent.
I feel lonely when I don't have plans for the weekend.
I feel withdrawn when I don't have anything to add to a conversation.

PRACTICE WITHOUT TRAINING WHEELS

Once you've practiced and practiced, you'll begin to feel like you really understand your sense of physical hunger. You will know the space when you feel satisfied and you can trust yourself to eat WHATEVER you want. Choosing your food without balancing your proteins and carbs would be fully following the principle of Intuitive Eating.

However, scientifically, keeping things balanced will help you satisfy your hunger, keep you full longer, your blood sugar stable and help you more clearly identify your fullness when it happens.[63]

It is harder to feel full when you've eaten nothing but carbs. So you might just recognize and acknowledge that you know that, but you are going to eat (fill in the blank) anyway. And leave out the guilt. If feeling guilty is a habit that's hard to break, try talking to yourself as if you were your own best friend.

Seriously, how would you respond to the negative comments being voiced in your head? We are usually more critical of ourselves than we would ever be of someone else. Treat yourself as a friend and trust yourself. That's the empowerment I'm talking about.

AND PRACTICE SOME MORE...

It can be frustrating to continually practice something that doesn't seem to get easier, especially if you are following ONE-TWO PUNCH for weight loss. It's easy to feel a little impatient. Or extremely impatient! When you're feeling down, let me remind you that you've already made a lot of progress. I know you have because you are reading this book and you're near the end!

Let me also remind you that there are all sorts of areas in your life that are going well. How do I know that? Because you at least had the motivation to get this book and read it, unless maybe you're a family member of mine and you're taking pity on me.

If we were visiting together in my office, I would be able to list all the ways you're rockin' it in multiple areas of your life. Eating is only one aspect of your life in which you need help.

I use the following analogy about practice and how it goes. Picture a basketball player — an amazing basketball player who is one of the starters on his team. He's an awesome, well-seasoned, diverse and talented athlete. Most games he racks up the most points. He has an excellent lay-up, he dribbles well and his 3-point shot is stellar. He's also a great team leader and his teammates respect and look up to him. What could be wrong, right?

He sucks at free throws. SUCKS! How can he have a stellar 3-point shot and suck at free throws? No clue. Maybe it's the pressure, the paused stance, the exact distance from the hoop. Who knows? But it's awful. It's become so bad the coach has to take him out of the game near the end so he doesn't get fouled. Other teams know his weakness too, so he's an easy target for fouling because they know he'll miss. It's a problem.

Does this make him less of an athlete? Some might argue yes, I'm well aware. I'll argue no, he just needs dedicated practice at free-throw shooting. Ding, ding, ding!!!

Wait, we are not done. So he commits to free-throw shooting practice every day with a designated coach. He shows up the first day and the coach gives him all kinds of pointers: how to stand, how the ball should feel in his hands, what to think, how to bend his knees, how the ball should leave his hands, the flexion of his wrists. He takes it all in, applies all the pointers and shoots. Nothing. Airball after airball after airball, with the occasional rim bounce, but still no shot. He gets nothing the entire practice.

Does he decide after that practice session that it just won't work? No! Although discouraged, he shows up the next day. And nothing again. Unbelievably discouraging! Determined, he shows up the day after that and tries again. And one time it goes in. He knew it would, he could feel it as the ball left his hands. He knew exactly how it felt and now he knew what to do to hear the quiet swish sound. Cool!!! Next shot – airball. Dammit (or for sure other expletives)! But one time, just one time, it had worked and he knew he could make it work again.

This is like your life. And I am your eating coach. You're rockin' it in many areas but can't seem to understand what it feels like to be truly physically hungry. It feels so foreign to you and seems so easy for other people. Combining a portion of protein and a portion of carb seems like a fairly simple concept, but sometimes you just don't want to.

Or, you're sick of doing it and your brain hurts from trying to figure out a combination that sounds appealing. Or you forget to apply what you've learned in this book. In those moments it seems so much easier to just follow a diet and eat exactly what you're told. It seems easier until it isn't. You can do this. There will be times that you nail it –

BOOMDIADA!! And other times you feel you miss the mark entirely.

    Remember there's no wagon to fall off of. You're not left in the dust and it doesn't mean you've blown it or even that you cheated. It just means your practice didn't go very well, or as well as you would have liked, for that particular meal. There's always the next meal. And the next time you get hungry. There are plenty of opportunities for practice to master the new skill and strike that knockout ONE-TWO PUNCH!

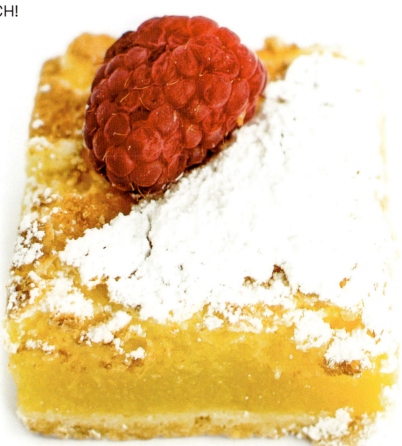

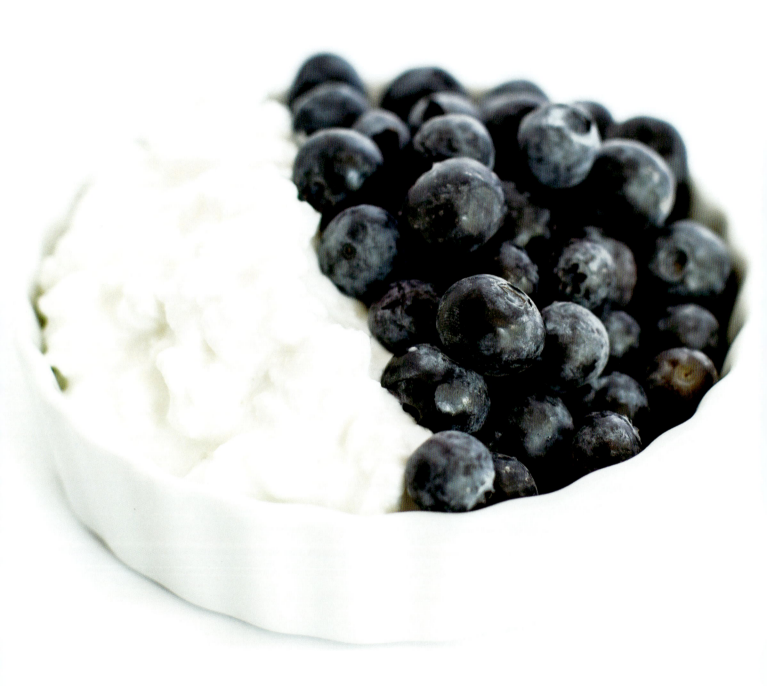

CONCLUSION

One-Two Punch

ONE-TWO PUNCH helps you:

- Be healthy and at the weight you want, without dieting.

- Lose weight without measuring your food, counting calories or recording your food intake.

- Eat what you want, without feeling deprived.

- Eat what your friends and family are eating.

- Balance your blood sugar.

- Stay full longer.

- Simplify your eating.

- Follow a program that is sustainable.

- Lose the guilt around eating and foods.

- Stop stressing about food.

Phew!!! You made it. ONE-TWO PUNCH was created to simplify eating, to take the stress out of it and bring enjoyment back. All while helping you achieve health and reach a weight you are comfortable with. Let's quickly summarize what we've been talking about.

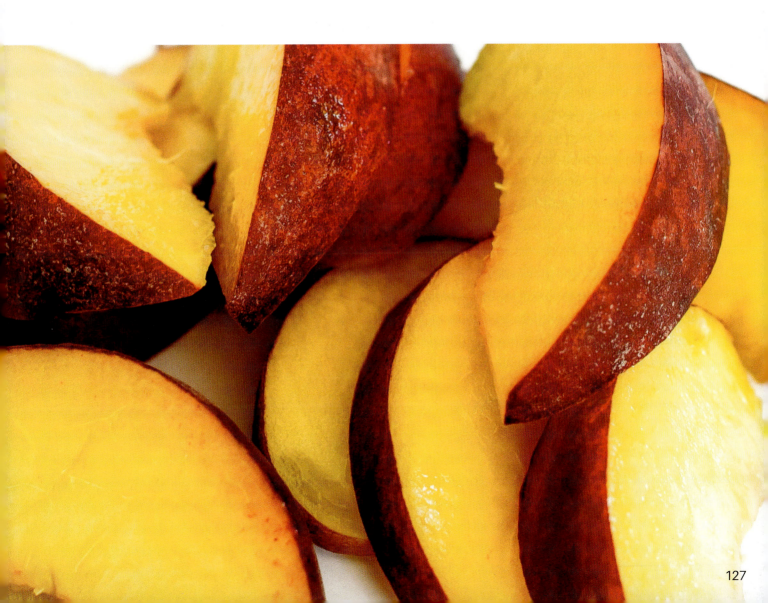

BURN

Respond when your body is hungry. Think of your stomach as an incinerator. When the incinerator door is open, when you're hungry, your body will BURN and use anything you put in it. When you feel hungry, it's your body's way of indicating you need fuel and it will BURN it.

As you eat, the incinerator door begins to close. Once closed, when your body signals that it is full, you have more potential for storing the extra food as fat. That happens when you eat past the point of fullness, but also when you eat when you're not hungry in the first place. So the first step is trying to eat only when you feel hungry.

BALANCE

Once you've determined that you are hungry, you need to BALANCE the protein and carbohydrate going into your incinerator to stabilize your blood sugar and to feel full longer. ONE-TWO PUNCH allows you to do this without measuring, counting or tracking by using the size of your fist. It's your "ONE-TWO PUNCH" towards health. The fist-size portion you choose can be any protein and any carbohydrate. It's your choice. That's the beauty of OTP — choices for days!

BECOME

Practice the process. It takes practice to decipher physical hunger from other emotions you might feel. It takes practice to estimate a fist-size portion of protein and a fist-size portion of carbohydrate when you eat. You need to practice choosing options of protein and carbohydrate that are most helpful to you in a particular circumstance. Practice is a verb – it's doing. Practice responding to your hunger. Practice sitting with feelings that are not hunger. Practice making different choices and determining how you feel. Practice trust. Practice forgiveness. Practice patience. Practice and then practice some more to become the YOU you've always wanted to be!

Eat when your body will **BURN** it
BALANCE what you eat
BECOME the YOU you've always wanted

This is a long-term, sustainable method for wellness. You can apply it ANYwhere, at ANY age, ANY ethnicity, ANY city, ANY country, ANY restaurant. It does take work and it does take commitment. As you practice this method, without overthinking it, you will be able to focus on the bigger issues like family, friends, relationships, work, health, your life. Respond to your body when it's going to BURN the food you give it, BALANCE your protein and carbohydrate every time you eat and this method will help you BECOME a healthy weight and have a healthy relationship with food.

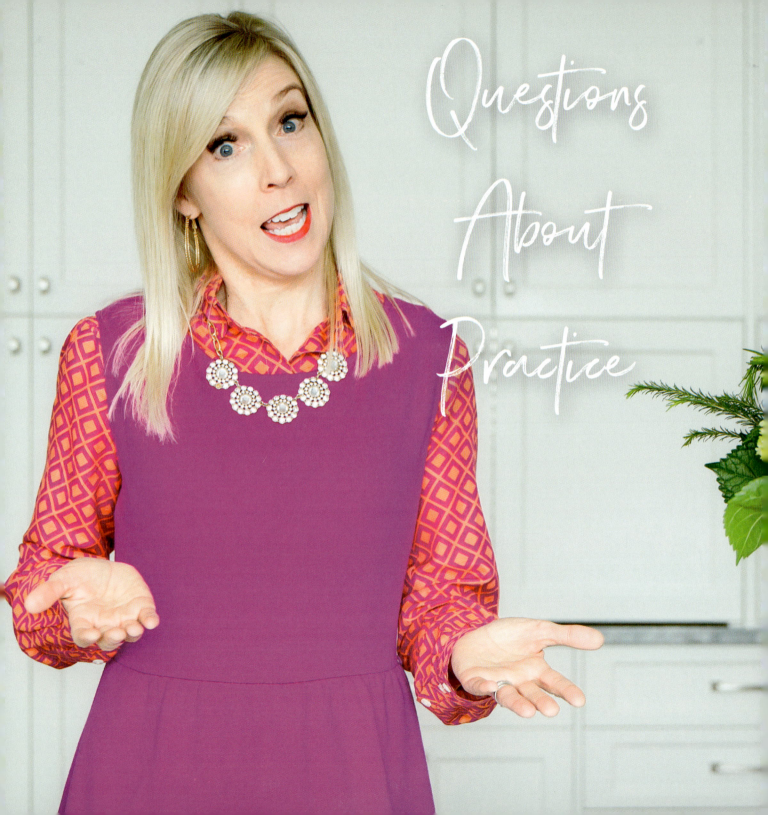

WHAT IF I'M STILL HUNGRY AFTER A BALANCED FIST-SIZED PORTIONS OF PROTEIN AND CARBOHYDRATE?

Make sure it has been 20-30 minutes since beginning to eat, to let your body communicate with your brain. Are you well hydrated? Did you include fat in your meal? It might be that you need more food.

If you are very active, it is possible that you will need more fuel (see next question). Try eating another balanced fist or try just a half-sized fist of each.

DO I NEED TO CHANGE THIS PLAN IF I EXERCISE?

One of the most beautiful things about ONE-TWO PUNCH is its simplicity. You do not need to recalculate anything, or calculate anything in the first place. Your physical hunger signals will adjust to your activity on their own. If you add extra activity into your day, you might find that you are hungry more often; this is your incinerator opening more often.

If you are strength training and aerobically exercising, you will have more muscle mass than if you are sedentary. Having more muscle mass increases your metabolism. When you have an increase in metabolism, you will feel more hungry and need to respond to that more often and eat more at each sitting to feel satisfied.

WHY ISN'T FAT COUNTED?

If you are using the guideline of a fist of protein and a fist of carbohydrate, it's going to be difficult to go crazy with fat to the extent that would be detrimental. Use fat as a condiment. Don't count the fat within your protein or carbohydrate choices or in what you add to your food, like butter, oil or salad dressings.

Added fat will only lead to increased physical and sensual satisfaction. Remember we're trying NOT to be too concerned with the details, just the general outline. Added fat will keep you full longer than having a low-fat combination of protein and carbohydrate. It all balances out when you eat for hunger and fullness.

WHEN SHOULD I HAVE BREAKFAST?

I hope after reading this book you can answer this question yourself! Yes, breakfast is important. It should be the first time you get hungry after you wake up; whenever that is for you. It might be first thing in the morning or not until you are showered and ready. It might even be after you get to work.

IS THERE A TIME THAT IS TOO LATE TO EAT?

I like to say "the carriage does not turn into a pumpkin" after a certain time of night. The reasons people lost weight after cutting off their eating after a certain time is because they were eating when they weren't hungry in the evening and eating more than their bodies needed. This is easy to do after a long day. They stopped that behavior and they lost weight. You can do that by only eating when you get hungry.

If you are truly physically hungry in the evening, you should eat. Remember that it's much more difficult to tell when you're tired. Look again at the hunger sequence chart.

WHAT'S THE DIFFERENCE BETWEEN A MEAL AND A SNACK?

Since the incinerator does not change in size, essentially we could say that there's no difference between the two — you eat when you're hungry, balance your protein and carbohydrate, then wait until the next time you get hungry to eat again. However, there might be a time that you don't want to get completely full.[87]

Let's say, for instance, that you have dinner plans at 7:00pm. It's 6:00pm and you are starving, ready to eat. If you fully satisfy yourself at this time, you won't be hungry when the rest of your group meets for dinner. You could have just enough pro/carb to take the edge off your hunger, so you can

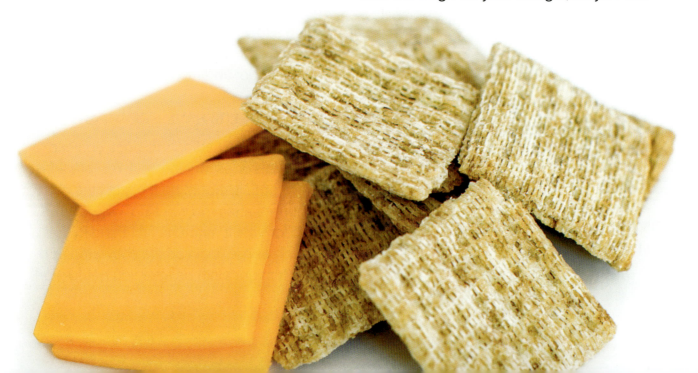

reasonably socialize and look over the menu, without getting completely full. I would call this a snack. Examples might be a glass of milk, a protein bar or half of it, half an apple with some nut butter and so on.

WHAT SHOULD I DO WHEN I EAT OUT?

You still follow ONE-TWO PUNCH. Choose a protein and choose a carbohydrate.

For instance, you are eating at an Italian restaurant and you want to have a pasta Alfredo dish. Your protein option to go with that dish might be chicken, but remember that it is a fist-size portion of pasta, not the heaping pile that is probably served to you. In addition, if bread was served before the entrée arrived, that is additional carbohydrate. If you really like the bread served as an appetizer then have it, but you might want to choose an entrée that has significantly fewer carbohydrates.

Regardless of the restaurant you choose, think of the Plate Builder, with a fist of your plate dedicated to protein and a fist of your plate dedicated to carbohydrates. Whether or not you add the vegetables, for the remaining half plate, is up to you.

WHAT IF I HATE VEGETABLES?

No problem. You can get around eating vegetables. Do they add fiber, vitamins, minerals, antioxidants to your meal and increase volume in your stomach to make you feel full? YES. But you can also have just a fist-size portion each of protein and carbohydrate without the vegetables. However, if you are not eating any vegetables, ever, I recommend taking a multivitamin-mineral supplement.

CAN I FOLLOW THIS METHOD IF I HAVE DIABETES?

Following ONE-TWO PUNCH is an excellent plan for people with diabetes, as it balances the foods going into your bloodstream and keeps your blood sugar from spiking. The protein and fat serve as anchors and slow down the carbohydrate entering your blood stream. It is the principle of never having an unaccompanied carbohydrate, and limiting the carbohydrate to a fist-size portion, that keeps the diabetes in check.

You might find after practicing this method that you don't need to count carbohydrates since you are controlling your portions by following the fist-size recommendation.

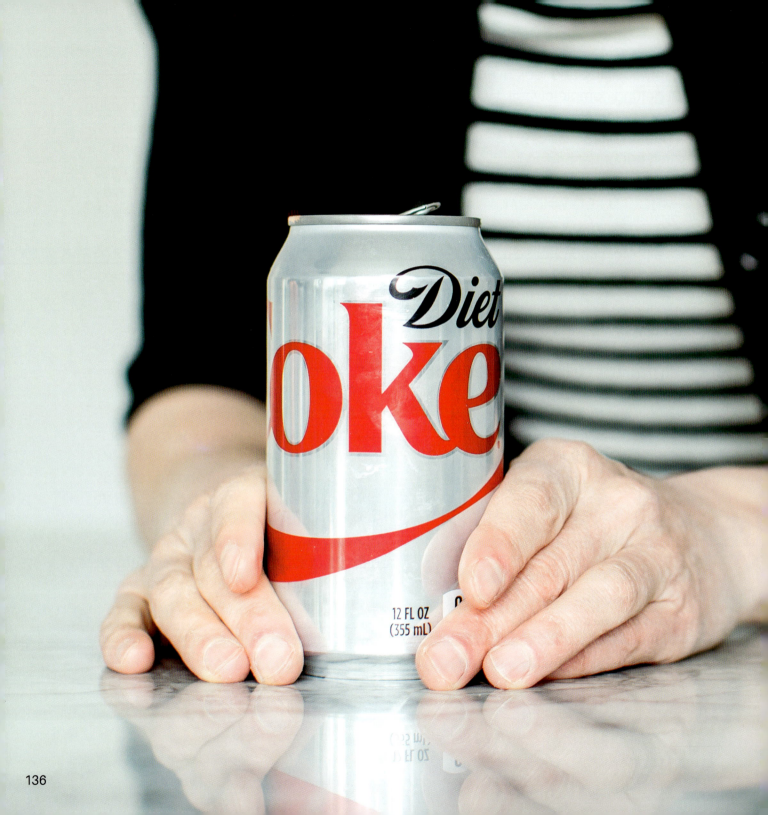

WHERE DOES DIET SODA FIT?

Any beverage without carbohydrates, or low in carbohydrates, can be added to a meal or snack without categorizing it as a protein, carb or fat. Sugary drinks are okay too, but you would need to categorize them as your fist of carbohydrate.

CAN I EAT WITH OTHER PEOPLE AND STILL PRACTICE MINDFUL EATING?

Yes. Eating with other people can certainly be distracting. It will be helpful to follow the guidelines in "Practice with Fullness" to pace your eating. Creating pause points to sense your fullness will help keep you focused.

HOW CAN I DO THIS WHILE TRAVELING?

ONE-TWO PUNCH can be done in any city, any country, any car, any airport, in any time zone. Remember the first foundational principle of BURN: eat when you are hungry and when your incinerator door is open. This applies while on vacation or business travel as well.

Yes, there are often excessive amounts of food available on vacation or at business lunches or dinners. Choose your fist-size portion of carbohydrate and your fist-size portion of protein from among those items.

WILL I LOSE WEIGHT WHILE FOLLOWING THIS?

If you were previously eating at times when not physically hungry and eating past the point of fullness, you will likely lose weight by eating only when physically hungry and portioning your food intake to a fistful each of protein and carbohydrate.

HOW IS THIS BETTER THAN INTUITIVE EATING?

Some people find that intuitive eating is too vague for them. The idea of eating anything they want when hungry, and even when they are not hungry, can be too abstract for some people. The process of becoming an intuitive eater is complex and takes time. ONE-TWO PUNCH offers some parameters and guidelines to eating, while still allowing for individual taste preferences and body awareness.

CAN I DO THIS WHILE TAKING MEDICATION?

Check with your doctor first regarding any foods that might interfere with a medication you are taking. In general, yes, this plan can be followed with most medications.

IS THIS OKAY TO DO WHILE PREGNANT OR NURSING?

Yes. Remember the first foundational principle of BURN: eat when you are hungry and when your incinerator door is open. If you are pregnant, you may find that you are hungry more often and that your taste preferences have changed. You can adjust ONE-TWO PUNCH accordingly, but it is still valuable to balance protein and carbohydrate.

The same rule applies to nursing. You may find that you are hungry more often while nursing and that it may take more than a fist each of protein and carbohydrate to feel full. Again, the plan can be adjusted accordingly.

SHOULD I WEIGH MYSELF WHILE DOING THIS? HOW OFTEN?

Weighing is a personal preference, but I don't recommend it. Here's why: You are practicing sensing your hunger and responding to it by having a balanced fist each of protein and carbohydrate.

You weigh yourself and your weight has decreased. You may think you can ease up on how careful you've been about distinguishing hunger and not pay as much attention. Or, you weigh yourself and your weight has stayed the same or increased. You may think that this doesn't work and that you need to go back to counting, tracking and measuring everything you eat in order to lose weight.

The bottom line: I think weighing "muddies the water" in our ability to focus on our hunger and fullness sensations. If you do decide to weigh yourself, I recommend no more than once per week.

WHAT IF I GAIN WEIGHT?

If you find that you are gaining weight with ONE-TWO PUNCH, there are several reasons for this. You may have needed to gain weight to be at an optimal weight for your body. It might be that you were previously ignoring hunger signals and now you are trying to respond to them. It might also take time for your body to become accustomed to you feeding it on a regular basis, throughout the day, as your hunger dictates.

It might be that you are mistaking what it feels like to be truly physically hungry. You might be thirsty or anxious and feeling something else besides physical hunger. If you are eating, even if it's a balanced protein and carb meal or snack, when the incinerator

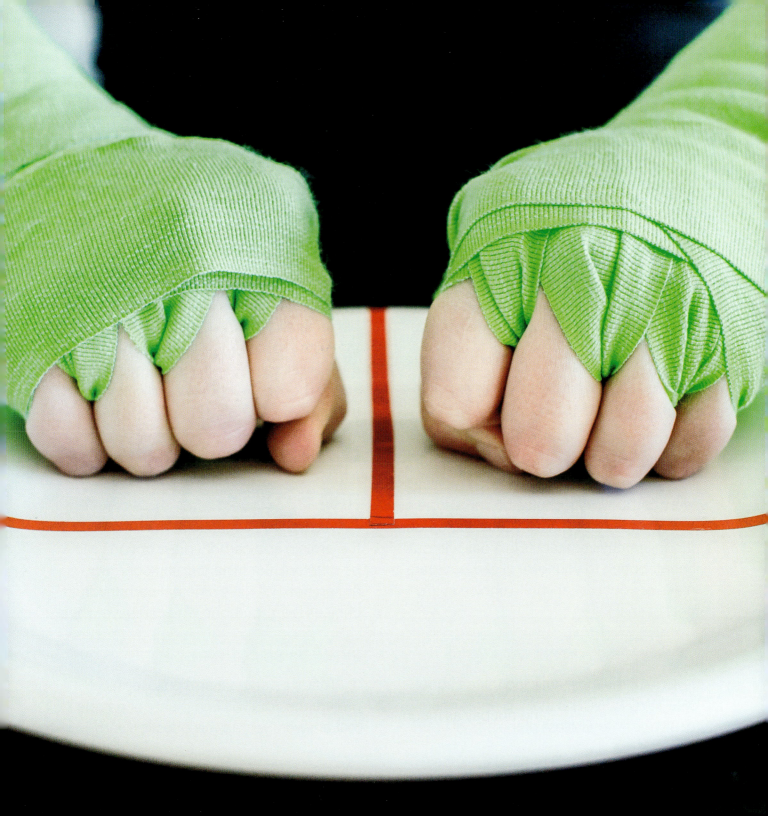

door is closed, you have more potential for weight gain.

WHAT SUPPLEMENTS AND VITAMINS SHOULD I TAKE?

If at least two of your carbohydrate choices per day are fruits and you are including half a plate of veggies at two or more meals or snacks, you probably don't need a multivitamin-mineral supplement. If, however, you don't like vegetables and most fruits, you may want to consider taking a supplement.

HOW MANY FRUITS AND VEGETABLES SHOULD I EAT DURING THE DAY?

A minimum intake, without adding a multivitamin-mineral supplement is listed above. However, you may choose to have every carbohydrate choice be some type of fruit. You may also have an unlimited amount of non-starchy vegetables in a day without it contributing to your overall carbohydrate intake or your carbohydrate choice at any meal or snack.

CAN MY KIDS DO THIS WITH ME?

One of the most amazing things about ONE-TWO PUNCH is that it is appropriate for all ages. Regardless of the age of your child or children, they can practice eating their own fist-size portion of protein and carbohydrate, and then more if they are still hungry. Young children are usually very good at distinguishing hunger and fullness cues. That ability sometimes fades as we age. Hopefully, your children will follow your example of practicing ONE-TWO PUNCH.

WHAT IF I AM VEGETARIAN OR VEGAN?

Both vegetarians and vegans can participate in ONE-TWO PUNCH. Of course, the protein options will be different, but there is still value in balancing the protein and carbohydrate choices and eating them together.

CAN I DO THIS TOGETHER WITH ANOTHER PLAN LIKE PALEO™ OR WHOLE30™?

Yes. As with vegetarians and vegans, the protein and carbohydrate options will be different. For instance, someone who is gluten-free will have different carbohydrate choices than someone who can have wheat.

SHOULD I BUY ORGANIC FOODS?

This is a personal and philosophical preference. You will find plenty of people that answer "yes" to this question and possibly an equal number of people that answer "no." Some people find that they feel better overall when they eat mostly organic foods. For some people, it's not feasible to eat mostly organic foods, either because of cost or because of the lack of availability of these foods in their area.

The focus of this book is guiding people to balance protein and carbohydrate when responding to hunger, regardless of what options might be available to them.

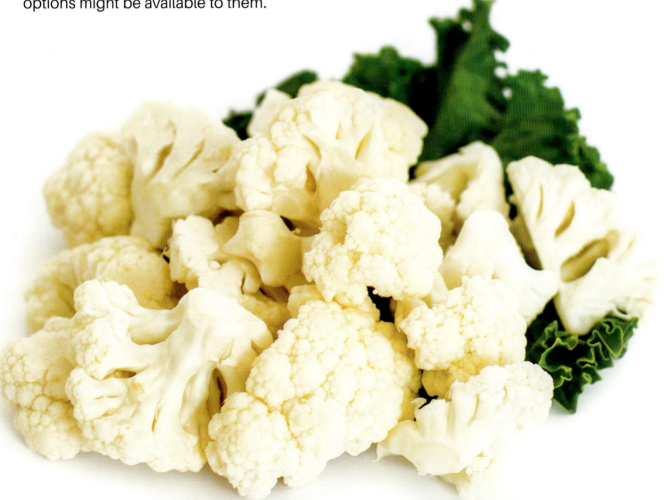

REFERENCES

1. 100 million dieters, $20 billion: The weight-loss industry by the numbers. Abc News. May 8, 2012.

2. Obesity and overweight. World Health Organization website.

3. Mozaffarian D, Benjamin E, Go A et al. Heart Disease and Stroke Statistics—2016 Update. Circulation. 2015;133(4):e38-e360.

4. Crabtree J. One third of the world is now obese or overweight but US adults aren't faring worst. CNBC June 14, 2017.

5. Tribole E, Resch E. Intuitive Eating: A Revolutionary Program That Works. 3rd ed. New York, NY: St. Martin's Press; 2012.

6. Tribole E. The difference between intuitive eating and mindful eating. Intuitive Eating website.

7. The Center for Mindful Eating. Why Mindful Eating?

8. Lofgren I. Mindful Eating. Am J Lifestyle Med. 2015;9(3):212-216.

9. Camilleri G, Méjean C, Bellisle F, Andreeva V, Kesse-Guyot E, Hercberg S, and Péneau S. Intuitive eating is inversely associated with body weight status in the general population-based NutriNet-Santé study. Obesity. 2016:24(5):1154–1161.

10. Tylka T. Development and psychometric evaluation of a measure of intuitive eating. J Couns Psycho. 2006: 53(2)226-240.

11. Bruce L, Ricciardelli L. A systematic review of the psychosocial correlates of intuitive eating among adult women. Appetite. 2016;96:454-472.

12. Herbert B, Blechert J, Hautzinger M, Matthias E, Herbert C. Intuitive eating is associated with interoceptive sensitivity. Effects on body mass index. Appetite. 2013;70:22-30.

13. Murray M, Vickers Z. Consumer views of hunger and fullness. A qualitative approach. Appetite. 2009;53(2):174-182.

14. Rebello C, Greenway F. Reward-Induced Eating: Therapeutic Approaches to Addressing Food Cravings. Adv Ther. 2016;33(11):1853-1866.

15. Moehlecke M, Canani L, Silva L, Trindade M, Friedman R, Leitão C. Determinants of body weight regulation in humans. Arch Endocrinol Metab. 2016;60(2):152-162.

16. Carson E. Pleasure overrides fullness when it comes to controlling food intake. SCAN's Pulse. 2016; 35(4):1-2.

17. Klok M, Jakobsdottir S, Drent M. The role of leptin and ghrelin in the regulation of food intake and body weight in humans: a review. Obes Rev. 2007;8(1):21-34.

18. Hayes M, Miller C, Ulbrecht J, Mauger J, Parker-Klees L, Gutschall M, Mitchell D, Smiciklas-Wright H, Covasa M. A carbohydrate-restricted diet alters gut peptides and adiposity signals in men and women with metabolic syndrome. J Nutr. 2007;137(8)1944-1950.

19. Power M, Schulkin J. Anticipatory physiological regulation in feeding biology: Cephalic phase responses. Appetite. 2008;50(2-3):194-206.

20. Zanchi D, Depoorter A, Egloff L et al. The impact of gut hormones on the neural circuit of appetite and satiety: A systematic review. Neurosci Biobehav Rev. 2017;80:457-475.

21. Suzuki K, Jayasena CN, Bloom SR. Obesity and Appetite Control. Experimental Diabetes Research. 2012;2012:824305.

22. Steen J. We found out if it really takes 20 minutes to feel full. Huffington Post Australia website.

23. Moran T. Gastrointestinal satiety signals II. Cholecystokinin. Am J Physiol Gastrointest Liver Physiol. 2004;286(2):183G-188.

24. Kolaczynski J. Response of leptin to short-term and prolonged overfeeding in humans. J Clin Endocrinol Metab. 1996;81(11):4162-4165.

25. Meinders AJ, Meinders AE. How much water do we really need to drink? Ned Tijdschr Geneeskd (Dutch). 2010;154:A1757.

26. Gropper S, Smith J, Groff J. Advanced Nutrition and Human Metabolism. 5th ed. Belmont, CA: Wadsworth; 2005: 299-300.

27. Perello M, Sakata I, Birnbaum S et al. Ghrelin Increases the Rewarding Value of High-Fat Diet in an Orexin-Dependent Manner. Biol Psychiatry. 2010;67(9):880-886.

28. Goldstone A, Prechtl C, Scholtz S et al. Ghrelin mimics fasting to enhance human hedonic, orbitofrontal cortex, and hippocampal responses to food. Am J Clin Nutr. 2014;99(6):1319-1330.

29. Gropper S, Smith J, Groff J. Advanced Nutrition and Human Metabolism. 5th ed. Belmont, CA: Wadsworth; 2005: 167-168.

30. MacDonald A. Why eating slowly may help you feel full faster. Harvard Health Publishing website.

31. Kokkinos A, le Roux C, Alexiadou K et al. Eating Slowly Increases the Postprandial Response of the Anorexigenic Gut Hormones, Peptide YY and Glucagon-Like Peptide-1. J Clin Endocrinol Metab. 2010;95(1):333-337.

32. Stroebe W, van Koningsbruggen G, Papies E, Aarts H. Why most dieters fail but some succeed: A goal conflict model of eating behavior. Psychol Rev. 2013;120(1):110-138.

33. Gropper S, Smith J, Groff J. Advanced Nutrition and Human Metabolism. 5th ed. Belmont, CA: Wadsworth; 2005: 251-254.

34. Berridge K. 'Liking' and 'wanting' food rewards: Brain substrates and roles in eating disorders. Physiol Behav. 2009;97(5):537-550.

35. Geiker N, Astrup A, Hjorth M, Sjödin A, Pijls L, Markus R. Does stress influence sleep patterns, food intake, weight gain, abdominal obesity and weight loss interventions and vice versa?. [Published online ahead of print August 28, 2017]. Obes Rev. 2018;19(1):81-97.

36. Tomiyama A, Mann T, Vinas D, Hunger J, DeJager J, Taylor S. Low Calorie Dieting Increases Cortisol. Psychosom Med. 2010;72(4):357-364.

37. Komaroff A. The gut-brain connection. Harvard Health Publishing website.

38. Loxton N, Dawe S, Cahill A. Does negative mood drive the urge to eat? The contribution of negative mood, exposure to food cues and eating style. Appetite. 2011;56(2):368-374.

39. Spence C, Okajima K, Cheok A, Petit O, Michel C. Eating with our eyes: From visual hunger to digital satiation. Brain Cogn. 2016;110:53-63.

40. Kroemer N, Krebs L, Kobiella A et al. (Still) longing for food: Insulin reactivity modulates response to food pictures. Hum Brain Mapp. 2012;34(10):2367-2380.

41. Cohen, D. Under the radar: What made you buy (and eat) that. Nutrition Action. 2016; March.

42. Vartanian L, Spanos S, Herman C, Polivy J. Conflicting internal and external eating cues: Impact on food intake and attributions. Health Psychol. 2017;36(4):365-369.

43. McHill A, Phillips A, Czeisler C et al. Later circadian timing of food intake is associated with increased body fat. Am J Clin Nutr. 2017;106(5):1213-1219.

44. Alexander K, Siegel H. Perceived hunger mediates the relationship between attachment anxiety and emotional eating. Eat Behav. 2013;14(3):374-377.

45. Dennis E, Dengo A, Comber D et al. Water consumption increases weight loss during a hypocaloric diet intervention in middle-aged and older adults. Obesity. 2009;18(2):300-307.

46. Mahan L, Escott-Stump S. Krause's Food and Nutrition Therapy. 12th ed. St. Louis, MO: Saunders Elsevier; 2008:147-148.

47. Duff R. Academy of Nutrition and Dietetics Complete Food and Nutrition Guide. 5th ed. Boston, NY: Houghton Mifflin Harcourt; 2017: 444-445.

48. An R, McCaffrey J. Plain water consumption in relation to energy intake and diet quality among US adults, 2005-2012. J Human Nutr Diet. 2016;29(5):624-632.

49. Popkin B, D'Anci K, Rosenberg I. Water, hydration, and health. Nutr Rev. 2010;68(8):439-458.

50. Muñoz C, Johnson E, McKenzie A et al. Habitual total water intake and dimensions of mood in healthy young women. Appetite. 2015;92:81-86.

51. Wöber C, Wöber-Bingöl Ç. Triggers of migraine and tension-type headache. Handb Clin Neurol. 2010:161-172.

52. Water & Nutrition. Centers for Disease Control and Prevention website.

53. Gonnissen H, Hursel R, Rutters F, Martens E, Westerterp-Plantenga M. Effects of sleep fragmentation on appetite and related hormone concentrations over 24 h in healthy men. Br J Nutr. 2012;109(04):748-756.

54. Spiegel K, Tasali E, Penev P, Van Cauter E. Brief communication: Sleep curtailment in healthy young men is associated with decreased leptin levels, elevated ghrelin levels, and increased hunger and appetite. Ann Intern Med. 2004;141(11):846-850.

55. Loxton N, Dawe S, Cahill A. Does negative mood drive the urge to eat? The contribution of negative mood, exposure to food cues and eating style. Appetite. 2011;56(2):368-374.

56. Bryant P, Trinder J, Curtis N. Sick and tired: does sleep have a vital role in the immune system? Nat Rev Immunol. 2004;4(6):457-467.

57. Chaput J, Klingenberg L, Sjödin A. Do all sedentary activities lead to weight gain: sleep does not. Curr Opin Clin Nutr Metab Care. 2010;13(6):601-607.

58. Greer S, Goldstein A, Walker M. The impact of sleep deprivation on food desire in the human brain. Nat Commun. 2013;4.

59. George R, Garcia A, Edwards C. Glycaemic responses of staple South Asian foods alone and combined with curried chicken as a mixed meal. J Hum Nutr Diet. 2014;28(3):283-291.

60. Hätönen K, Virtamo J, Eriksson J, Sinkko H, Sundvall J, Valsta L. Protein and fat modify the glycaemic and insulinaemic responses to a mashed potato-based meal. Br J Nutr. 2011;106(02):248-253.

61. Gropper S, Smith J, Groff J. Advanced Nutrition and Human Metabolism. 5th ed. Belmont, CA: Wadsworth; 2005: 14,74-75.

62. Chang K, Lampe J, Schwarz Y et al. Low glycemic load experimental diet more satiating than high glycemic load diet. Nutr Canc. 2012;64(5):666-673.

63. Bellissimo N, Akhavan T. Effect of Macronutrient Composition on Short-Term Food Intake and Weight Loss. Adv Nutr. 2015;6(3):302S-308S.

64. Hosseinpour-Niazi S, Sohrab G, Asghari G, Mirmiran P, Moslehi N, Azizi F. Dietary glycemic index, glycemic load, and cardiovascular disease risk factors: Tehran Lipid and Glucose Study. Arch Iran Med. 2013;16(7):401-407.

65. Dhillon J, Craig B, Leidy H et al. The Effects of Increased Protein Intake on Fullness: A Meta-Analysis and Its Limitations. J Acad Nutr Diet. 2016;116(6):968-983.

66. Gropper S, Smith J, Groff J. Advanced Nutrition and Human Metabolism. 5th ed. Belmont, CA: Wadsworth; 2005: 300.

67. Mozaffarian D. Foods, obesity, and diabetes—are all calories created equal? Nutr Rev. 2017;75(suppl 1):19-31.

68. Dhillon J, Craig B, Leidy H et al. The Effects of Increased Protein Intake on Fullness: A Meta-Analysis and Its Limitations. J Acad Nutr Diet. 2016;116(6):968-983.

69. Maki KC, Rains TM, Kaden VN, Raneri KR, Davidson MH. Effects of a reduced-glycemic-load diet on body weight, body composition, and cardiovascular disease risk markers in overweight and obese adults. Am J Clin Nutr. 2007;85(3):724-734.

70. Sofer S, Stark A, Madar Z. Nutrition Targeting by Food Timing: Time-Related Dietary Approaches to Combat Obesity and Metabolic Syndrome. Adv Nutr. 2015;6(2):214-223.

71. Gibson A, Hsu M, Rangan A et al. Accuracy of hands v. household measures as portion size estimation aids. J Nutr Sci. 2016;5.

72. vanDellen M, Isherwood J, Delose J. How do people define moderation?. Appetite. 2016;101:156-162.

73. Duff R. Academy of Nutrition and Dietetics Complete Food and Nutrition Guide. 5th ed. Boston, NY: Houghton Mifflin Harcourt; 2017: 359-361.

74. Duff R. Academy of Nutrition and Dietetics Complete Food and Nutrition Guide. 5th ed. Boston, NY: Houghton Mifflin Harcourt; 2017: 381.

75. Grodner M, Escott-Stump S. Nutritional Foundations and Clinical Applications: A Nursing Approach. 6th ed. St. Louis, MO: Elsevier Mosby; 2016.

76. Byrne S, Cooper Z, Fairburn C. Psychological predictors of weight regain in obesity. Behav Res Ther. 2004;42(11):1341-1356.

77. Kuijer R, Boyce J. Chocolate cake. Guilt or celebration? Associations with healthy eating attitudes, perceived behavioural control, intentions and weight-loss. Appetite. 2014;74:48-54.

78. Mozaffarian D. Dietary and Policy Priorities for Cardiovascular Disease, Diabetes, and Obesity. Circulation. 2016;133(2):187-225.

79. Pollan M. In Defense of Food: An Eater's Manifesto. New York, NY: Penguin Books; 2008.

80. Linardon J, Mitchell S. Rigid dietary control, flexible dietary control, and intuitive eating: Evidence for their differential relationship to disordered eating and body image concerns. Eat Behav. 2017;26:16-22.

81. Tribole E, Resch E. Intuitive Eating: A Revolutionary Program That Works. 3rd ed. New York, NY: St. Martin's Press; 2012: 220.

82. MIT Medical. Hunger scale. https://medical.mit.edu/sites/default/files/hunger_scale.pdf.

83. Omichinski L. You Count, Calories Don't. London, UK: Hodder & Stoughton; 1996.

84. Doğan T, Tekin E, Katrancıoğlu A. Feeding your feelings: A self-report measure of emotional eating. Procedia Soc Behav Sci. 2011;15:2074-2077.

85. Andrade A, Greene G, Melanson K. Eating Slowly Led to Decreases in Energy Intake within Meals in Healthy Women. J Am Diet Assoc. 2008;108(7):1186-1191.

86. Shah M, Copeland J, Dart L, Adams-Huet B, James A, Rhea D. Slower eating speed lowers energy intake in normal-weight but not overweight/obese subjects. J Acad Nutr Diet. 2014;114(3):393-402.

87. Ogden J, Wood C, Payne E, Fouracre H, Lammyman F. 'Snack' versus 'meal': The impact of label and place on food intake. Appetite. 2018;120:666-672.

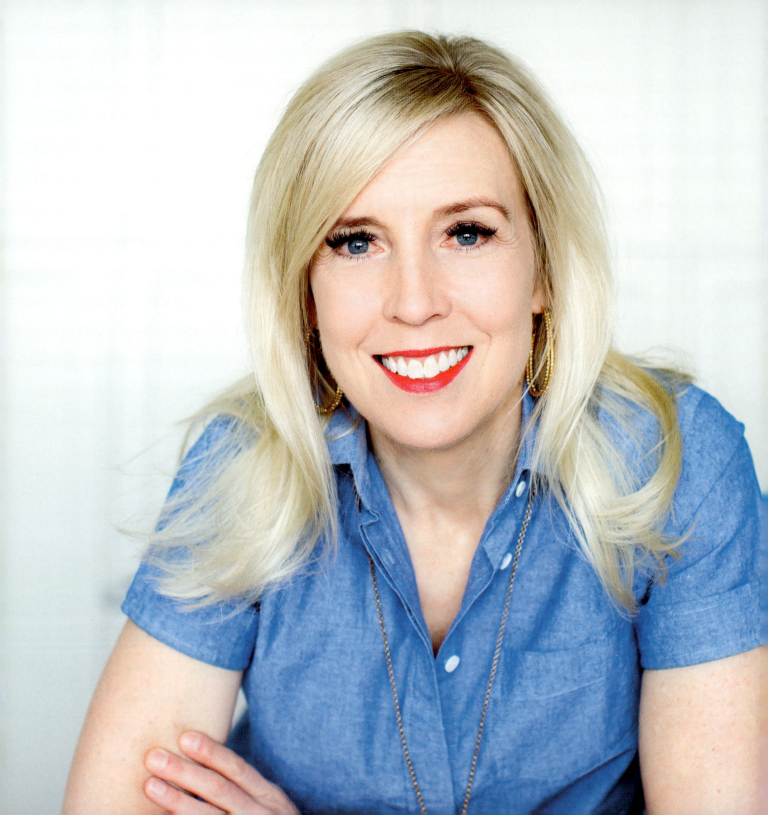

ABOUT CLAUDIA

Claudia Wilson is the owner and founder of ALL of NUTRITION and creator of ONE-TWO PUNCH™. She is passionate about helping clients have it ALL by simplifying. Claudia helps clients examine all the areas in their lives that affect their eating and nutrition. Together they work to bring about balance in the body and in life. In that sense, she acts as a life coach, but more specifically an EATING COACH.

In private practice, she works with clients and organizations on a variety of issues including general wellness, sports nutrition, eating disorders, intuitive eating, weight management, diabetes, allergies and intolerances, high cholesterol, healthy eating, meal planning and other issues related to nutrition.

She is a Registered Dietitian Nutritionist, certified in the state of Utah and a Board Certified Specialist in Sports Nutrition (CSSD). She is also a Strength and Conditioning Specialist/Trainer (CSCS). She received her Bachelor's Degree in Public Health from West Chester University in Pennsylvania and her Master's Degree in Nutrition from the University of Utah, with an emphasis in Sports Nutrition and Eating Disorders.

Claudia spent nearly 10 years as a sports nutritionist with the University of Utah Athletic Department, serving all female and male athletic teams, and the Department of Family and Preventive Medicine as a clinical dietitian nutritionist. She has served on the U.S. Gatorade Nutrition Advisory Board and Speaker Network. She is currently a member of the Academy for Nutrition and Dietetics (AND), Sports, Cardiovascular, and Wellness Nutritionists (SCAN) and the National Strength and Conditioning Association (NSCA).

ACKNOWLEDGEMENTS

One definition of brigade is a fleet of trained people. That is absolutely what I had; a posse of hugely talented individuals that helped make this happen! An enormous thank you to the following:

Andrew and Jessi Adams of Strom Communications. In addition to much needed comic relief, Andrew for his marketing genius and all things IT. Jessi for being graphic designer extraordinaire, complete with the never-ending patience to work with me and calm that makes the whole world a better place.

Partner at All of Nutrition, Marysa Cardwell, for her fresh perspective and intellect. She, together with Andrea Walsh, our stellar intern, are research masterminds.

Lindsay Salazar Photography for the beautiful photos. Nearly all of the photos in the book are her work.

Marti Grace Ashby and Ali Spencer for reading, editing and taking me seriously.

And finally, my family...you guys put up with SO much! Thank you for appeasing me and for your priceless input.